Agnessa Kozak

Muskel-Skelett-Erkrankungen und Beschwerden bei Beschäftigten in Gesundheits- und Pflegeberufen

Kumulative Dissertation zu Häufigkeiten,
Risiken und Interventionsmöglichkeiten

Agnessa Kozak

Muskel-Skelett-Erkrankungen und Beschwerden bei Beschäftigten in Gesundheits- und Pflegeberufen

Kumulative Dissertation zu Häufigkeiten,
Risiken und Interventionsmöglichkeiten

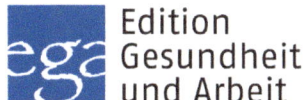
Edition
Gesundheit
und Arbeit

© 2017
Edition Gesundheit und Arbeit,
Schriftenreihe des CVcare, Band 7

Muskel-Skelett-Erkrankungen und Beschwerden
bei Beschäftigten in Gesundheits- und Pflegeberufen

Kumulative Dissertation zu Häufigkeiten,
Risiken und Interventionsmöglichkeiten

Universitätsklinikum Hamburg-Eppendorf (UKE),
CVcare | Bethanien-Höfe Eppendorf
Martinistraße 52, 20246 Hamburg
www.uke.de

Herausgeber
Prof. Dr. med. Albert Nienhaus
a.nienhaus@uke.de

Autor
Agnessa Kozak

Redaktion
Elisabeth Muth

Lektorat
Angelika Buchholz, Frankfurt

Gestaltung
Ethel Knop

Verlag
tredition GmbH, Hamburg
ISBN: 978-3-7323-8678-9

Printed in Germany

Bibliografische Information der Deutschen Nationalbibliothek
Die Deutsche Nationalbibliothek verzeichnet diese Publikation in der Deutschen Nationalbibliografie; detaillierte bibliografische Daten sind im Internet über http://dnb.d-nb.de abrufbar.

Inhaltsverzeichnis

Vorwort Herausgeber

Die Edition Gesundheit und Arbeit (ega) ist eine Schriftenreihe des Competenzzentrums für Epidemiologie und Versorgungsforschung bei Pflegeberufen (CVcare) am Universitätsklinikum Hamburg-Eppendorf (UKE).

Mit der *ega* soll die Diskussion im deutschsprachigen Raum über effektive und effiziente Wege zur Verbesserung des Gesundheitsschutzes, der betrieblichen Gesundheitsförderung sowie des betrieblichen Gesundheitsmanagements unter besonderer Berücksichtigung der betrieblichen Wiedereingliederung sowie der Rehabilitation gefördert werden. Die *ega* ist eine Plattform für interdisziplinäre Beiträge aus der arbeitsweltbezogenen Gesundheitsforschung. Die Disziplinen Psychologie, Arbeitsmedizin, Gesundheitswissenschaften, Gesundheitsökonomie, Rehabilitations- und Versorgungsforschung sollen damit näher zusammengeführt und zum gegenseitigen Austausch angeregt werden.

Das CVcare ist eine universitäre Forschungseinrichtung am UKE, deren Grundfinanzierung durch eine Stiftung der Berufsgenossenschaft für Gesundheitsdienst und Wohlfahrtspflege (BGW) sichergestellt wird. Das CVcare kooperiert daher eng mit der BGW und hier insbesondere mit deren Forschungsbereich Grundlagen der Prävention und Rehabilitation (GPR).

Das CVcare stellt epidemiologische Daten zur Arbeits- und Gesundheitssituation von Pflegekräften und anderen Beschäftigten im Gesundheitswesen und in der Wohlfahrtspflege zur Verfügung. Angebote zur arbeitsweltbezogenen Gesundheitsförderung, Prävention und Rehabilitation werden unter besonderer Berücksichtigung des demografischen Wandels im Sinne der Versorgungsforschung überprüft. In praxisorientierten Projekten werden Vorschläge zur eventuellen Verbesserung dieser Angebote entwickelt.

Schwerpunktthemen des CVcare sind die Arbeitssituation älterer Beschäftigter in der Pflege, arbeitsbedingte Beschwerden des Bewegungsapparates (MSB), Infektionsrisiken mit den Schwerpunkten Tuberkulose und multiresistente Erreger (MRE), psychosoziale Belastungen am Arbeitsplatz mit dem besonderen Schwerpunkt Gewalt am Arbeitsplatz sowie die Evaluation der Rehabilitationsleistungen der BGW und anderer Träger der gesetzlichen Unfallversicherung (GUV).

Der siebte Band der Edition gibt die PhD-Arbeit „Muskel-Skelett-Erkrankungen und Beschwerden bei Beschäftigten in Gesundheits- und Pflegeberufen" von Agnessa Kozak wieder. In einem Methodenmix bestehend aus Befragung, Meta-Analyse und Interventionsstudie belegt Agnessa Kozak in ihrer kumulativen Arbeit, dass Muskel-Skelett-Erkrankungen und Beschwerden (MSE/MSB) bei Tierärzten und Auszubildenden in der Pflege häufig auftreten und mit beruflichen Belastungen assoziiert sind. Für das Carpaltunnel-Syndrom (CTS) arbeitet sie die beruflichen Risikofaktoren heraus und liefert damit eine verbesserte Grundlage zur Beurteilung des CTS als Berufskrankheit. In ihrer Interventionsstudie zeigt sie, dass ungünstige Körperhaltungen in der Pflege durch ergonomische und edukative Maßnahmen deutlich reduziert werden können und liefert so einen wichtigen Ansatz zur Prävention von MSE/MSB.

Die PhD-Arbeit wurde von Prof. Dr. Gabriele Perger von der Hochschule für angewandte Wissenschaften (HAW) und Prof. Dr. Monika Bullinger vom Institut für medizinische Psychologie am UKE betreut. Dafür möchte ich mich an dieser Stelle bei beiden Hochschullehrerinnen herzlich bedanken.

Es freut mich, dem interessierten Leser die facettenreiche, methodisch anspruchsvolle und anwendungsorientierte Arbeit zu berufsbedingten MSE/MSB von Agnessa Kozak in der Schriftenreihe *ega* zur Verfügung stellen zu können.

Hamburg, im Februar 2017   Prof. Dr. med. Albert Nienhaus

Publikationsliste

Kozak A[1], Schedlbauer G[2], Peters C[1], Nienhaus A[1,2] (2014)

Self-Reported Musculoskeletal Disorders of the Distal Upper Extremities and the Neck in German Veterinarians: A Cross-Sectional Study.
PLOS ONE 9(2): e89362

[1] Institut für Versorgungsforschung in der Dermatologie und bei Pflegeberufen,
Universitätsklinikum Hamburg-Eppendorf

[2] Berufsgenossenschaft für Gesundheitsdienst und Wohlfahrtspflege,
Abteilung Grundlagen der Prävention und Rehabilitation

Wirth T[1], Kozak A[2], Schedlbauer G[1], Nienhaus A[1,2] (2016)

Health Behaviour, Health Status and Occupational Prospects of Apprentice Nurses and Kindergarten Teachers in Germany: A Cross-Sectional Study.
J Occup Med Toxicol 11(26)

[1] Berufsgenossenschaft für Gesundheitsdienst und Wohlfahrtspflege,
Abteilung Grundlagen der Prävention und Rehabilitation

[2] Institut für Versorgungsforschung in der Dermatologie und bei Pflegeberufen,
Universitätsklinikum Hamburg-Eppendorf

Kozak A[1], Schedlbauer G[2], Wirth T[2], Euler U[3], Westermann C[1], Nienhaus A[1,2] (2015)

Association between Work-Related Biomechanical Risk Factors and the Occurrence of Carpal Tunnel Syndrome: An Overview of Systematic Reviews and a Meta-Analysis of Current Research.
BMC Musculoskel Dis 16(231)

[1] Institut für Versorgungsforschung in der Dermatologie und bei Pflegeberufen,
Universitätsklinikum Hamburg-Eppendorf

[2] Berufsgenossenschaft für Gesundheitsdienst und Wohlfahrtspflege,
Abteilung Grundlagen der Prävention und Rehabilitation

[3] Institut und Poliklinik für Arbeits- und Sozialmedizin, Technische Universität Dresden

Kozak A[1], Freitag S[2], Nienhaus A[1,2] (2017)

Evaluation of a Training Program to Reduce Stressful Trunk Postures in the Nursing Professions: A Pilot Study.
Annals of Work Exposures and Health 61(1)

[1] Institut für Versorgungsforschung in der Dermatologie und bei Pflegeberufen,
Universitätsklinikum Hamburg-Eppendorf

[2] Berufsgenossenschaft für Gesundheitsdienst und Wohlfahrtspflege,
Abteilung Grundlagen der Prävention und Rehabilitation

Die deutsche Übersetzung der ersten drei Studien wurden in Buchbeiträgen des Ecomed Verlags veröffentlicht. Es ist eine Aufsatzsammlung von kooperierenden Forschungsprojekten der BGW, des CVcare und weiterer Forschungseinrichtungen:

RiRe – Risiken und Ressourcen in Gesundheitsdienst und Wohlfahrtspflege. Band 1 (2014) und Band 2 (2015), Nienhaus, A. (Hrsg.), ecomed: Landsberg am Lech.

1 Abstracts

Publikation 1

Muskuloskelettale Beschwerden der oberen Extremitäten und des Nackens bei Veterinären in Deutschland – eine Querschnittsstudie

Hintergrund: Muskuloskelettale Beschwerden (MSB) sind eine bedeutsame Gesundheitsstörung bei praktizierenden Veterinären. Zwangshaltungen, repetitive Tätigkeiten, schweres Heben und Tragen und von Tieren verursachte Unfälle sind häufige Risikofaktoren für MSB, insbesondere der oberen Extremitäten. In der vorliegenden Studie werden die 12-Monats-Prävalenz von MSB, die Häufigkeit der daraus resultierenden funktionellen Einschränkungen dargestellt sowie die Häufigkeit der arbeitsbedingten Unfälle, die MSB zur Folge hatten. Darüber hinaus wird untersucht, welche Faktoren mit einer Beschwerdelast der oberen Extremitäten in Zusammenhang stehen.

Methode: An der 2011 durchgeführten fragebogenbasierten Prävalenzstudie nahmen 3.174 Veterinäre (Responserate: 38,4%) aus sieben Kammerbezirken teil. Die Teilnehmer wurden zu MSB, den tierärztlichen Tätigkeiten sowie zu ihrer psychomentalen Verfassung befragt. Verwendet wurde der standardisierte Nordic Questionnaire und Teile aus dem Copenhagen Psychosocial Questionnaire.

Ergebnisse: MSB am Nacken (66,6%) und an der Schulter (60,5%) wurden häufiger genannt als an der Hand (34,5%) oder am Ellenbogen (24,5%). Diese Beschwerden führten zu Einschränkungen im Alltag: Hals (28,7%), Schulter (29,5%), Hand (19,4%) und Ellbogen (14%). Die 12-Monats-Prävalenz von MSB der distalen oberen Extremitäten war bei Großtierpraktikern signifikant höher als bei den übrigen Tierärzten. Dagegen klagten vor allem Kleintierpraktiker über Beschwerden im Nacken. Von Unfällen, die MSB zur Folge hatten, waren am häufigsten die Hand (14,3%) oder die Schulter (10,8%) betroffen. Die meisten Unfälle, die den Oberkörper verletzten, gingen von Tieren aus (19% vs. 9,2%). Je nach Körperregion trugen persönliche und arbeitsbedingte Faktoren wesentlich zur Beschwerdelast bei: höheres Alter, Geschlecht, frühere Verletzungen, BMI, Praxistyp, häufig durchgeführte veterinäre Tätigkeiten wie Zahnmedizin, rektale Untersuchungen und Geburtshilfe sowie hohe Anforderungen und Burnout.

Schlussfolgerungen: Erstmals konnte gezeigt werden, dass MSB bei Tierärzten in Deutschland häufig auftreten. Maßnahmen zur Prävention von belastenden Körperhaltungen und Bewegungen sowie Unfällen erscheinen sinnvoll und notwendig. Bei der Implementierung von Maßnahmen sollten der Praxistyp, geschlechtsspezifische sowie psychosoziale Faktoren berücksichtigt werden.

Publikation 2

Gesundheitsverhalten, Gesundheitszustand und Zukunftsperspektiven von Auszubildenden in pflegerischen und sozialen Berufen – eine Querschnittsstudie

Hintergrund: Im Dienstleistungssektor des Gesundheits- und Sozialwesens sind Beschäftigte hohen emotionalen und körperlichen Belastungen ausgesetzt. Dementsprechend fällt der Bereich durch hohe Arbeitsunfähigkeits- und Berufsaussteigerquoten auf. Die Ausbildungsphase bietet einzigartige Möglichkeiten, frühzeitig durch Vermittlung gesundheitsfördernder Verhaltensweisen zu intervenieren. Das Ziel dieser Arbeit ist es, den Gesundheitszustand, das Gesundheitsverhalten sowie Zukunftsperspektiven von Auszubildenden in pflegerischen und sozialen Berufen vergleichend darzustellen sowie Faktoren im Zusammenhang mit ihrer körperlichen und psychischen Gesundheit zu identifizieren.

Methoden: Von Januar bis März 2014 wurde eine fragebogenbasierte Querschnittsstudie an acht Hamburger Berufsschulen der Altenpflege, Gesundheits- und Krankenpflege, Erziehung und sozialpädagogischen Assistenz durchgeführt. Unterschiede zwischen den Ausbildungsberufen wurden mittels Chi^2-Tests und Varianzanalysen ermittelt. Anhand von logistischen Regressionsanalysen wurden gesundheitsbezogene Faktoren auf ihren Zusammenhang mit körperlichen und psychischen Erkrankungen geprüft.

Ergebnisse: 402 Auszubildende nahmen an der Befragung teil (Responserate: 99%). In der Altenpflege sowie in der Erziehung und sozialpädagogischen Assistenz waren knapp 33% der Befragten übergewichtig oder adipös. 55% der Auszubildenden in der Altenpflege rauchten. Die Arbeitszufriedenheit war am geringsten bei den Auszubildenden in der Gesundheits- und Krankenpflege. Mehr als ein Drittel der Befragten litt an muskuloskelettalen und psychischen Beschwerden. Auszubildende zwischen dem 23. und 26. Lebensjahr und solche, die psychisch beeinträchtigt waren, hatten eine höhere Wahrscheinlichkeit für muskuloskelettale Beschwerden (OR 3,1, 95%-KI 1,4–6,7 beziehungsweise OR 1,8, 95%-KI 1,1–3,1). Auszubildende in sozialen Berufen wiesen eine höhere Wahrscheinlichkeit auf für psychische Beeinträchtigungen im Vergleich zu Auszubildenden in anderen Berufen. Ebenfalls zeigte sich, dass geringe Selbstwirksamkeit und hohe Irritation mit erhöhten psychischen Beeinträchtigungen im Zusammenhang standen.

Schlussfolgerungen: Die Ergebnisse der Arbeit verdeutlichen, dass berufsgruppenübergreifend Handlungsbedarf zur Förderung eines nachhaltigen Gesundheitsverhaltens in Berufsschulen besteht. Insbesondere Auszubildende in der Altenpflege könnten von präventiven Maßnahmen profitieren. Aufgabe zukünftiger Forschungsprojekte sollte sein, erfolgreiche Konzepte und Maßnahmen zu entwickeln und zu evaluieren, um die Gesundheit der Auszubildenden frühzeitig zu fördern und zu erhalten.

Publikation 3

Zusammenhang zwischen berufsbedingten Belastungsfaktoren und Karpaltunnelsyndrom – eine Übersichtsarbeit über systematische Reviews und eine Meta-Analyse aktueller Studien

Hintergrund: Das Karpaltunnelsyndrom (KTS) wird durch eine Kompression des Nervus medianus im Karpaltunnel verursacht. In den vergangenen Jahren wurden mehrere systematische Reviews zur Verursachung von KTS durch arbeitsbedingte biomechanische Belastungsfaktoren publiziert und das KTS wurde in die Liste der Berufskrankheiten aufgenommen. Das Ziel dieser Arbeit ist eine systematische Zusammenfassung und inhaltliche Bewertung dieser Studien, um die bis zum jetzigen Zeitpunkt bestehende Evidenz darzustellen.

Methoden: In den Datenbanken MEDLINE, EMBASE, CINAHL und Cochrane Library wurde systematisch nach Reviews gesucht, die seit 1998 publiziert wurden. Die Qualitätsbewertung wurde mit dem AMSTAR-R vorgenommen. Der Überschneidungsgrad von Originalarbeiten in den Reviews wurde mittels Corrected Covered Area (CCA) ermittelt. Im zweiten Schritt wurden Primärstudien gesucht, die seit 2011 publiziert wurden. Ihre methodologische Qualität wurde mit einem 20 Items umfassenden Instrument bewertet. Die Bewertung der Evidenz erfolgte qualitativ entsprechend der methodischen Qualität und Aktualität der Studien sowie der Konsistenz der Ergebnisse. Auf der Basis der aktuellen Primärstudien wurde eine Meta-Analyse zur Bestimmung der Dosis-Wirkung-Beziehungen durchgeführt.

Ergebnisse: Zehn systematische Reviews wurden eingeschlossen, die 143 Originalarbeiten berücksichtigten. Der CCA-Wert lag bei 13,3% und deutet auf einen hohen Grad der Überschneidung hin. Sieben aktuelle Primärstudien wurden identifiziert; vier davon waren Längsschnittuntersuchungen. Es besteht eine hohe Qualität der Evidenz für die Beziehung zwischen Repetition, Kraftaufwand sowie kombinierte Belastungen und KTS. Die Qualität der Evidenz für Vibration ist als moderat und für nicht neutrale Handpositionen als gering einzuschätzen. Eine Verursachung von KTS durch Computerarbeit ist aus epidemiologischer Perspektive unwahrscheinlich. Basierend auf den Aktivitätsgraden der ACGIH, zeigt die Meta-Analyse, dass kombinierte Belastungen oberhalb des Aktionslimits (bedenkliche Gefährdung) ein erhöhtes Risiko für KTS darstellen (RR 1,5; 95%-KI 1,02–2,31); oberhalb des Schwellenlimits (Gefährdung) verdoppelt sich das Risiko (RR 2,0; 95%-KI 1,46–2,82).

Schlussfolgerungen: Eine berufliche Verursachung durch Repetition, Kraftaufwand und kombinierte Belastungen ist sehr wahrscheinlich; Vibration kann das Risiko erhöhen, wenn sie über einen längeren Zeitraum andauert. Chronische Flexion und Extensionshaltungen bei der Arbeit können wahrscheinlich in Kombination mit anderen Faktoren das Risiko erhöhen. Die Verursachung von KTS durch PC-Arbeit ist unzureichend gesichert. Daten aus aktuellen Primärstudien deuten auf eine Dosis-Wirkung-Beziehung zwischen kombinierten Belastungsfaktoren und KTS hin.

Publikation 4

Messtechnische Evaluation eines Seminars zur Reduktion und Vermeidung von ungünstigen Körperhaltungen bei Altenpflegekräften

Hintergrund: In der vorliegenden Studie wurde die Wirksamkeit eines Basisseminars zur Reduzierung von ungünstigen Körperhaltungen im Arbeitsalltag bei Altenpflegekräften messtechnisch evaluiert.

Methode: Auf zwölf geriatrischen Stationen in sechs Altenpflegeheimen wurde ein zweitägiges Basisseminar durchgeführt mit dem Ziel, die Altenpflegekräfte für die körperlichen Belastungen während der Arbeit zu sensibilisieren und Möglichkeiten zur alternativen Ausführung ihrer Tätigkeiten mit weniger ungünstigen Körperhaltungen aufzuzeigen. Mit dem personengebundenen CUELA-Messsystem wurden alle Oberkörperneigungen vor und sechs Monate nach dem Seminar messtechnisch erfasst. Es wurden insgesamt 23 Frühschichten gemessen. Die Probanden wurden mit einer Videokamera über die gesamte Schicht begleitet. Mithilfe einer speziell entwickelten Software konnten die Messdaten und Videoaufnahmen synchronisiert werden.

Ergebnisse: Der mediane Zeitanteil in sagittalen Neigungen über 20° wurde sechs Monate nach der Intervention um 29% signifikant reduziert (von 35,4% Interquartilsabstand (27,6–43,1) zu 25,3% (20,7–34,1); P<0,001). Stark ausgeprägte Rumpfneigungen von mehr als 60° (2,5% (1,1–4,6) zu 1,0% (0,8–1,7); P=0,002) und statische Körperhaltungen über 20° und länger als 4 Sekunden (4,4% (3,0–6,7) zu 3,6% (2,5–4,5); P<0,001) wurden um 60% beziehungsweise 22% verringert. Videoanalysen zeigten, dass in 49% der Pflegesituationen die gelernten Arbeitsmethoden am Bett und im Bad richtig angewandt wurden.

Schlussfolgerung: Es wurde gezeigt, dass durch relativ geringen organisatorischen Aufwand und durch Informationsvermittlung ungünstige Körperhaltungen in der Altenpflege verringert werden konnten. Die konsequente Anpassung von höhenverstellbaren Betten oder die ergonomische Umgestaltung von Bewohnerzimmern kann maßgeblich dazu beitragen, die vielen belastenden Körperhaltungen zu reduzieren.

2 Synopse

Diese kumulative Arbeit trägt zum besseren Verständnis von arbeitsbezogenen und branchenspezifischen biomechanischen Belastungen bei Beschäftigten in Gesundheits- und Pflegeberufen bei, die zu Muskel-Skelett-Beschwerden (MSB) beziehungsweise zu -Erkrankungen (MSE) führen können. Im Fokus stehen die Ursachenforschung sowie die Verhütung dieser Beschwerden und Erkrankungen.

Die Zusammenhänge zwischen arbeitsbezogenen Belastungen und der Entwicklung von MSE/MSB werden seitens der einzelnen akademischen Disziplinen, der Öffentlichkeit oder der Versicherungsträger unterschiedlich beurteilt. Beispielsweise verlässt sich die klassische Orthopädie bei der Beurteilung von MSE auf morphologisch nachweisbare Störungen der Struktur und Funktionen, während die Ergonomie auch die psychosozialen und organisationsbedingten Bezüge zu MSE herstellt. Aus Sicht der Versicherungsträger stehen zum Beispiel medizinisch-statistische Größen wie Arbeitsunfähigkeit oder Feststellung einer Berufserkrankung (BK) im Vordergrund. Die Epidemiologie wiederum untersucht die Häufigkeiten, Indikatoren und ihre Beziehungen untereinander zur Bewertung der Relevanz bekannter Zusammenhänge in bestimmten Bevölkerungs- beziehungsweise Berufsgruppen sowie zur Generierung von Hypothesen über neue Phänomene (Hartmann & Spallek 2009). In der vorliegenden Arbeit werden epidemiologische Herangehensweisen angewandt, um eine Gesamtschau der Erkenntnisse für bestimmte Berufs- und Qualifikationsprofile zu skizzieren und Entscheidungsvorschläge für die Bewertung und Prävention von MSE/MSB zu generieren. Das Ziel dieser Arbeit besteht darin, themen- beziehungsweise berufsgruppengebunden auf bestehende Problemsituationen im Zusammenhang mit MSE/MSB hinzuweisen sowie Empfehlungen bereitzustellen. Im Rahmen dieser kumulativen Dissertation wird erstmalig aufgezeigt, wie häufig MSB bei Veterinärmedizinern in Deutschland vorkommen und welche Faktoren damit im Zusammenhang stehen. Eine weitere empirische Arbeit untersucht Gesundheitsverhalten, -zustand und Zukunftsperspektiven von Auszubildenden in pflegerischen und sozialen Berufen. Anhand einer systematischen Literaturarbeit wird dargestellt, welche berufsbedingten biomechanischen Belastungsfaktoren zur Entstehung eines Karpaltunnelsyndroms beitragen. Schließlich werden die Evaluationsergebnisse eines Schulungskonzeptes zur Reduzierung von ungünstigen Körperhaltungen in der Altenpflege vorgestellt, die mit einem personengebundenen Messsystem erfasst wurden.

Erkenntnisse über die Beziehung zwischen berufsbezogenen Faktoren und Erkrankungen sind die Handlungsbasis für Unfallversicherungsträger bei der Prävention von Gesundheitsgefahren sowie der Feststellung und Anerkennung von BKen. Gemäß dem gesetzlichen Auftrag sind Unfallversicherungsträger verpflichtet, Arbeitsunfälle, BKen und arbeitsbedingte Gesundheitsgefahren zu verhüten (§ 14, Abs. 1 SGB VII) sowie rehabilitative Leistungen im Versicherungsfall sicherzustellen (§ 11 SGB VII). Darüber hinaus sind sie verpflichtet, an den Forschungsvorhaben zur Fortentwicklung des BK-Rechts mitzuwirken und diese zu fördern (§ 9 Abs. 8 SGB VII). Insofern ist diese kumulative Dissertation im Rahmen von Teilprojekten entstanden, die durch die Arbeitsgruppe MSE innerhalb der Abteilung Grundlagen der Prävention und Rehabilitation bei der Berufsgenossenschaft für Gesundheitsdienst und Wohlfahrtspflege (BGW) initiiert und koordiniert wurden. Die Fragestellungen ergaben sich zum einen aus der Beratungstätigkeit sowie der Qualitätssicherung bei BK-Begutachtungsverfahren von Versicherten und zum anderen aus Anregungen der Selbstverwaltung der BGW. Seit 2010 fördert die BGW eine Stiftungsprofessur am Universitätsklinikum Hamburg-Eppendorf, die eigenständige und unabhängige Forschung im Bereich der arbeitsweltbezogenen Gesundheitsförderung, Prävention und Rehabilitation betreibt. Es besteht also eine enge Kooperation zwischen der BGW und dem Competenzzentrum Epidemiologie und Versorgungsforschung bei Pflegeberufen (CVcare). Forschungsschwerpunkt am CVcare ist die Untersuchung von risikobelasteten berufsbezogenen Tätigkeiten, die Interaktion dieser Risikofaktoren untereinander sowie die Erarbeitung von gezielten Präventions- und Rehabilitationsmaßnahmen. Die Bandbreite der Beschwerdebilder, ihre Pathomechanismen sowie Präventionsmaßnahmen von beziehungsweise gegen berufsbezogene(n) MSE sind ebenso vielfältig wie die methodischen Herangehensweisen zur Analyse dieser Beschwerdebilder und Maßnahmen. Außerdem besteht Forschungsbedarf für spezielle Berufs- und Qualifikationsprofile im Gesundheits- und Sozialsektor in Deutschland. Einleitend wird zunächst die MSE/MSB-bedingte Krankheitslast vorgestellt. Daran anknüpfend wird die berufliche Verursachung von MSE/MSB bei Beschäftigten in Gesundheits- und Pflegeberufen veranschaulicht. In diesem Abschnitt werden epidemiologische und arbeitsmedizinische Erkenntnisse jeweils für die einzelnen Studienzielsetzungen differenziert begründet und diese anschließend für jede Studie formuliert. Methodische Herangehensweisen, Ergebnispräsentation sowie Diskussion der Ergebnisse werden ebenfalls für jede Studie separat herausgearbeitet.

2.1 Hintergrund

Muskel-Skelett-Erkrankungen gehören zu den häufigsten Leiden in der deutschen Bevölkerung. Sie nehmen im Durchschnitt den größten Anteil an Arbeitsunfähigkeitstagen (AU-Tage) in den AU-Statistiken der gesetzlichen Krankenversicherungen ein. Für das Jahr 2014 ging geschlechtsübergreifend knapp ein Viertel aller AU-Tage auf MSE zurück, da diese häufig mit langen Ausfallzeiten verbunden waren (DAK 2015; Meyer et al. 2015; TK 2015). In dieser Diagnosehauptgruppe (ICD-10: M00-M99) stellten Rückenerkrankungen mit insgesamt 44% den größten Anteil an AU-Tagen dar (Meyer et al. 2015). Nach psychischen Störungen (50%) waren MSE der häufigste Grund (13%) für eine vorzeitige Erwerbsunfähigkeit im Jahr 2014 (DRV 2015). Dementsprechend verursachen MSE hohe direkte und indirekte volkswirtschaftliche Kosten. Von den insgesamt 103 Milliarden Euro Verlust an Bruttowertschöpfung durch Arbeitsunfähigkeit im Jahr 2013 entfielen 22,7 Milliarden Euro allein auf Krankheiten des Bewegungsapparates (BAuA 2015). Nicht zuletzt resultieren daraus hohe intangible Kosten für die Betroffenen, wie körperliche Funktionseinschränkungen, chronische Schmerzen oder Verlust an Lebensqualität (Picavet & Hoeymans 2004; Roux et al. 2005). Der Global-Burden-of-Disease-Studie zufolge nehmen MSE, gemessen in Disability-Adjusted Life Years (DALY), bei Frauen den ersten und bei Männern den dritten Rang der Krankheitslast ein. Im Zeitraum von 1990 bis 2010 sind die absoluten DALYs für Rückenschmerzen um 11% gestiegen; sie sind damit auch im internationalen Vergleich die häufigste Ursache für die Krankheitslast (Plass et al. 2014).

Obwohl die Ursachen von MSE/MSB komplex sind und multiple Faktoren diese bedingen (Balague et al. 2012), ist ihre berufliche Verursachung von besonderer Relevanz. In epidemiologischen Studien ist hinreichend belegt, dass MSE durch berufsspezifische physikalische, physische und psychomentale Einwirkungen und damit zusammenhängende Über- und Fehlbelastung des Haltungs- und Bewegungsapparates verursacht werden (Bernard 1997; Ochsmann & Winkler 2009). Insbesondere die Tätigkeiten im Gesundheits- und Pflegesektor können je nach Häufigkeit, Dauer und Intensität der belastenden Faktoren die verschiedenen Strukturen des Bewegungsapparates (z. B. Knochen, Sehnen, Muskeln, Nerven) beanspruchen. Die Erkrankungen und Beschwerdebilder haben einen heterogenen Charakter; sie unterscheiden sich je nach Lokalisation[1] und der betroffenen Gewebsstruktur erheblich voneinander (Hoehne-

---

[1] Die Beschwerden werden nach ihrer Lokalisation unterschieden: obere Extremitäten und Halswirbelsäule (HWS, C1-C7), Brustwirbelsäule (BWS, Th1-Th12) und Lendenwirbelsäule (LWS, L1-L5) sowie untere Extremitäten. In der vorliegenden Arbeit wird der Fokus auf obere Extremitäten und Rücken (HWS und LWS) gerichtet.

Hückstädt et al. 2007). Im aktuellen DAK-Gesundheitsreport wird für den Wirtschaftszweig „Gesundheitswesen" der höchste Krankenstand von 4,5% angegeben (DAK 2015). Dieser hohe Krankenstand ist sowohl auf eine überdurchschnittliche Erkrankungshäufigkeit als auch auf eine überdurchschnittliche Dauer der AU-Fälle zurückzuführen. Beispielsweise weisen Beschäftigte in der Altenpflege mit 25,7 AU-Tagen die zweitlängste AU-Dauer je Versicherungsjahr (TK 2013) auf. Erkrankungen an der Wirbelsäule zählen zu den häufigsten Leiden in dieser Berufsgruppe, doch auch Erkrankungen der oberen Extremitäten werden beobachtet. Zum Beispiel zeigt eine berufsbezogene Analyse von aggregierten Krankenkassendaten, dass bei der Berufsgruppe „Helferinnen in der Krankenpflege" 19.307 AU-Fälle in der Diagnosegruppe „Rückenschmerzen (M45)" und 1.524 AU-Fälle in der Diagnosegruppe „Mononeuropathie der oberen Extremität (G56)" gemeldet wurden (Liebers & Caffier 2009). Analog dazu legt die Statistik der BGW dar, dass die meisten Verdachtsmeldungen auf bandscheibenbedingte Erkrankungen der Lendenwirbelsäule (BK 2108) aus Altenpflege- und Altenkrankenheimen (31,8%) oder aus Krankenhäusern und Kliniken stammen (31,8%) (Wendeler et al. 2015). Die Ergebnisse der AU-, Unfall- und Reha-Statistiken verdeutlichen, warum die meisten Forschungsarbeiten den Fokus auf die Ursachenforschung und Prävention von Gesundheitsrisiken in der Pflege legen. Epidemiologische Untersuchungen zeigen ebenfalls, dass Pflegekräfte durchschnittlich häufiger über Rückenschmerzen berichten (12-Monats-Prävalenzrate 55%) (Davis & Kotowski 2015) als die Allgemeinbevölkerung (39%) (Hoy et al. 2012). Diese hohe Erkrankungs- beziehungsweise Symptomprävalenz in pflegerischen Berufen erklärt sich zum einen durch große körperliche Anstrengung und zum anderen auch durch psychosoziale Arbeitsbelastungen. Dazu zählen vor allem die Transfers und Mobilisation von Patienten (Engkvist et al. 2000; Eriksen et al. 2004; Pompeii et al. 2009), sagittale Neigungen des Oberkörpers in Kombination mit Hebe- und Tragevorgängen (Holtermann et al. 2013) sowie statische und erzwungene Haltungen (da Costa & Vieira 2010; Hodder et al. 2010). Weitere Faktoren wie unregelmäßige und lange Arbeitszeiten (Caruso & Waters 2008) sowie ein inadäquater Personalschlüssel (Kim et al. 2014) beeinflussen die körperliche Leistungsfähigkeit zusätzlich. Nicht zuletzt nimmt auch das psychosoziale Arbeitsumfeld Einfluss auf die Entwicklung von MSE/MSB (Lang et al. 2012). Einer aktuellen Meta-Analyse zufolge stehen geringer Handlungsspielraum, geringe soziale Unterstützung sowie ein Ungleichgewicht zwischen Anstrengung und Gegenleistung (Effort-Reward Imbalance) in einem signifikanten Zusammenhang mit MSB in verschiedenen Körperregionen bei Krankenpflegern und Krankenpflegehelfern (Bernal et al. 2015).

Strukturelle und gesellschaftliche Veränderungen können ebenfalls einen Einfluss auf die Arbeitssituation von Beschäftigten in Gesundheits- und Pflegeberufen nehmen. Die Entwicklungsdynamik in der Pflege und dabei insbesondere im Altenpflegesektor lässt vermuten, dass die körperlichen und psychischen Anstrengungen in den kommenden Jahren noch weiter zunehmen werden. Zum einen wird deutlich, dass der steigende Bedarf an Pflegefachkräften bereits jetzt spürbar ist und noch weiter zunehmen wird. Wird der Rückgang des Erwerbspersonenpotenzials bei gleichzeitig bundesweitem Anstieg der pflegebedürftigen Menschen berücksichtigt (um circa 47% im Jahr 2030), so steigt der Bedarf auf annähernd eine halbe Million Vollzeitäquivalente für das Jahr 2030 (Rothgang et al. 2012). Auch die demografische Struktur innerhalb des Pflegesektors wird sich verändern. Bereits heute sind mehr als die Hälfte der Alten- (62%) sowie Gesundheits- und Krankenpflegekräfte (59%) älter als 40 Jahre (DESTATIS 2015). Mit steigendem Alter nimmt die Anzahl und Schwere degenerativer Erkrankungen zu (Coggon et al. 2013; de Zwart et al. 1995). Folglich ist mit einer verminderten Leistungs- beziehungsweise Arbeitsfähigkeit (Camerino et al. 2006) sowie mit häufigen und längeren AU-Zeiten zu rechnen (Liebers et al. 2013). Zum anderen steigt die Komplexität aufgrund von Finanzierungsproblemen, unklaren Ausbildungsregelungen sowie zunehmender Bürokratisierung (Behr 2015).

Eine eingehende Darstellung und Analyse der MSE und ihrer Gesundheitsrisiken in den einzelnen Gesundheits- und Pflegeberufen würde den Rahmen dieser Arbeit sprengen, da sowohl die Erkrankungsarten als auch die Gesundheitsberufe heterogen sind. Nachfolgend wird also für jede Fragestellung dieser kumulativen Arbeit der theoretische Hintergrund umrisshaft dargestellt.

2.1.1 Berufsbedingte Risiken bei Veterinären

Veterinärmediziner zählen zu einer Berufsgruppe mit vielfältigen und häufigen berufsbedingten Risiken. Studien mit praktizierenden Veterinären zeigen, dass die tierärztliche Tätigkeit sowohl körperlich als auch psychisch belastend ist (Harling et al. 2009; Loomans et al. 2008; Reijula et al. 2003) und große Risiken für Erkrankungen und Unfälle mit zum Teil schwerwiegenden Verletzungen birgt (Fritschi et al. 2006; Lucas et al. 2009; Nienhaus et al. 2005). Die Routinedaten der BGW für den Zeitraum von 2007 bis 2011 verdeutlichen, dass die Tiere die häufigste Ursache für einen meldepflichtigen Arbeitsunfall sind (78%) (Kozak et al. 2012). Insbesondere die Versorgung von Großtieren geht mit MSE und MSB der oberen Extremitäten einher.

Bei Untersuchungen und Behandlungen neigen Tiere zu Abwehrreaktionen, die zu Verletzungen führen können (Abbildung 1) (Berry et al. 2012; Cattell 2000). Des Weiteren sehen Veterinäre die manuelle Handhabung von Tieren und Ausrüstung, rektale Untersuchungen sowie chirurgische Eingriffe als risikobehaftete Tätigkeiten für MSB und MSE an (Scuffham et al. 2010a). Diese und weitere Tätigkeiten erfordern häufig statische oder ungünstige Körperhaltungen sowie Repetition und Kraftaufwand. Durch die wiederholte Überbeanspruchung der oberen Extremitäten können Mikrotraumata entstehen, die auch als „Repetitive Strain Injuries" (RSI) oder „Cumulative Trauma Disorders" (CTD) bezeichnet werden[2]. Im Vergleich zu Allgemeinärzten und ihren Beschäftigten ist das Risiko für Beschäftigte in der Veterinärpraxis um den Faktor 2,9 erhöht (Nienhaus et al. 2005). Die immanenten Eigenschaften dieses Tätigkeitsfeldes können demnach zur erhöhten Prävalenz von MSB-Symptomen beitragen, die sich in funktionellen Beeinträchtigungen und/oder schlimmstenfalls in chronischen Erkrankungen des Bewegungsapparates äußern.

Anlass für diese Untersuchung waren mehrere Fälle von Großtierpraktikern, die unter Erkrankungen im Bereich der oberen Extremitäten litten und ein Berufskrankheitsverfahren bei der BGW eingeleitet haben. Die Anerkennung als BK ist allerdings schwierig, denn der Zusammenhang zwischen der beruflichen Tätigkeit als Tierarzt und den Erkrankungen der oberen Extremitäten ist nicht hinreichend belegt. Zudem lagen bisher für Deutschland keine Daten zur Beschwerdehäufigkeit für diese Berufsgruppe vor. Auch ein möglicher Zusammenhang zwischen der Arbeitssituation und MSB ist bei dieser Berufsgruppe wenig erforscht.

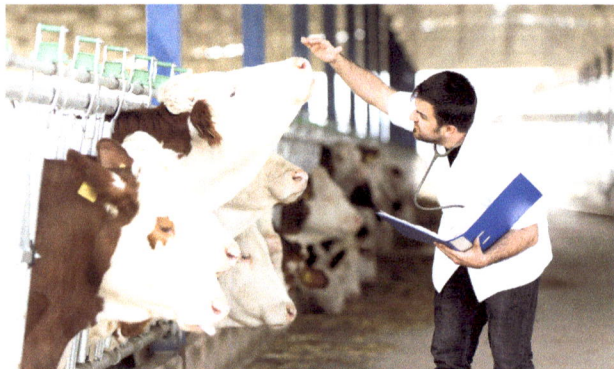

Abbildung 1 Veterinärmedizinische Untersuchung in einem Rinderstall

---

[2] Es handelt sich um Symptome und Krankheitsbilder mit zum Teil heterogenem Charakter, die durch entzündliche und degenerative Prozesse Schmerzen und Funktionsstörungen an Sehnen, Muskeln und Nerven verursachen.

2.1.2 Gesundheitszustand, -verhalten und Perspektiven von Auszubildenden in pflegerischen und sozialen Berufen

Der Bedarf und die Anzahl an Fachkräften in Sozial-und Gesundheitsberufen ist zum einen durch den demografischen Wandel und zum anderen durch den Ausbau der Infrastruktur für die Kinderbetreuung in den letzten Jahren erheblich gestiegen (Dathe et al. 2012). Wie eingangs beschrieben, sind Tätigkeiten im pflegerischen Bereich mit vielfältigen berufsbezogenen Belastungen verbunden. Die Arbeitsbedingungen im sozialen Bereich, insbesondere in Kindertagesstätten sind durch einen dauerhaft hohen Geräuschpegel und häufiges Arbeiten in gebeugter und gedrehter Körperhaltung gekennzeichnet. Dies kann zu psychischen und muskuloskelettalen Beschwerden führen (Almstadt et al. 2012; Koch et al. 2015).

Bereits Auszubildende sind diesen vielfältigen körperlichen und psychischen Arbeitsbelastungen ausgesetzt. Hinzu kommt, dass Auszubildende sich in einem Prozess des Erwachsenwerdens befinden und in dieser Phase besonders empfänglich für Reize ungesunder Lebensführung sind (Kaminski et al. 2008; Remschmidt 2013). Bisherige nationale und internationale Studienergebnisse verdeutlichen, dass Auszubildende in Pflegeberufen häufig einen gesundheitsgefährdenden Lebensstil aufweisen. Dies zeigt sich insbesondere durch den häufigen Konsum von Fast-Food-Produkten (Lindeman et al. 2011; Purcell et al. 2006; Schwanke et al. 2011), hohen Raucherquoten (in Deutschland teilweise über 50%) (Hirsch et al. 2010; Kolleck 2004; Neumann & Klewer 2010) sowie riskantem Trinkverhalten (Hirsch et al. 2010; Watson et al. 2006). Darüber hinaus sind Übergewicht und Adipositas bei Auszubildenden in der Pflege (Purcell et al. 2006; Singleton et al. 2011) und bei Beschäftigten in Erziehungsberufen (Baldwin et al. 2007; Hoffmann et al. 2013) stark verbreitet.

Auszubildende in Sozial-und Gesundheitsberufen berichten bereits von beruflich bedingten Belastungsfolgen wie Muskel-Skelett-Beschwerden und Erkrankungen sowie psychischen Beeinträchtigungen wie Depression oder Burnout (Crary 2013; Hausmann 2009; Mitchell et al. 2009). In diesen Berufszweigen werden außerdem hohe Arbeitsunfähigkeits- und Berufsaussteigerquoten beobachtet (Almstadt et al. 2012; Glaser & Höge 2005).

In früheren Studien zum Gesundheitszustand und -verhalten von Auszubildenden wurde nicht zwischen den verschiedenen Fachdisziplinen differenziert (z. B.

Gesundheits- und Krankenpflege sowie Altenpflege); dies erscheint jedoch sinnvoll, da die gesundheitlichen Belastungen in der Gesundheits- und Krankenpflege möglicherweise geringer ausfallen als in der Altenpflege (Simon et al. 2005). Außerdem soll geklärt werden, ob sich solche Unterschiede bereits in der Ausbildung zeigen. Darüber hinaus gibt es kaum Literatur zum Gesundheitszustand und -verhalten von Auszubildenden aus dem Bereich der Sozialen Arbeit. Zudem wurde ein Großteil der bisherigen Studien mit Auszubildenden in Sozial- und Gesundheitsberufen überwiegend im Ausland durchgeführt. Es ist anzunehmen, dass die Ergebnisse aufgrund unterschiedlicher Ausbildungssysteme nur eingeschränkt auf Deutschland übertragbar sind. Im Gegensatz zum Lehrlingsausbildungssystem in Deutschland wurde die Ausbildung in anderen europäischen Ländern akademisiert (Rudman & Gustavsson 2012; Timmins et al. 2011).

2.1.3 Biomechanische Faktoren als Ursache für ein Karpaltunnel-syndrom

Beim Karpaltunnelsyndrom (KTS) handelt es sich pathophysiologisch um eine periphere Mononeuropathie, die durch eine Erhöhung des Gewebsdrucks im Karpaltunnel hervorgerufen wird. In der Folge kommt es zu Druckschädigungen des Nervus medianus, verbunden mit sensorischen und motorischen Ausfällen im betroffenen Areal (Abbildung 2). KTS ist das häufigste Kompressionssyndrom eines peripheren Nervs (Assmus et al. 2007). Je nach Diagnosekriterien, Population oder Studientyp variiert die KTS-Prävalenz zwischen 0,6 und 61% (Hagberg et al. 1992).

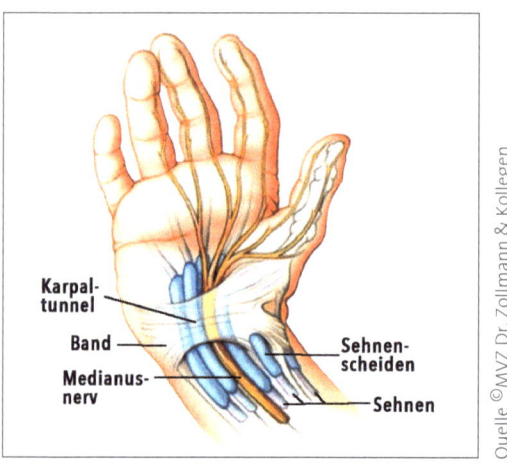

Abbildung 2 Knöcherne und straffe fibröse Begrenzung im Karpaltunnel

Die Ursachen für ein KTS können lokal (z. B. Zysten), regional (z. B. rheumatoide Arthritis) oder systemisch (z. B. Diabetes) bedingt sein (Aroori & Spence 2008). In der Literatur wird zunehmend belegt, dass die Entwicklung eines KTS durch repetitive Tätigkeiten mit Beugung und Streckung der Hände, erhöhtem Kraftaufwand oder Vibrationsbelastung begünstigt werden kann (Bernard 1997; Hagberg et al. 1992). Bestimmte Berufsgruppen sind durch ihre Tätigkeiten stärker exponiert als andere. Vorwiegend handelt es sich um Berufe mit häufiger Nutzung von handgehaltenen, vibrierenden Geräten und manuellen Anforderungen, insbesondere in der Montagearbeit und Lebensmittelverarbeitung beziehungsweise -verpackung (Palmer et al. 2007). Da KTS in der Allgemeinbevölkerung häufig vorkommt und die Ursachen multikausal sind, stellt sich die Frage, welchen Anteil arbeitsbezogene Faktoren insbesondere bei Beschäftigten im Gesundheitssektor ausmachen.

Ursprünglich wurde angestrebt, ursächliche Faktoren für KTS und ihre Interaktion untereinander bei Beschäftigten in Gesundheits- und Pflegeberufen auf Basis von epidemiologischen Studien zu untersuchen mit dem Ziel, konkrete Expositionsangaben für diese Berufsgruppen zu erarbeiten. Die erste systematische Literatursuche ergab, dass zu dem damaligen Zeitpunkt kaum qualitativ robuste Studien vorlagen. Überwiegend handelte es sich um Querschnittsstudien, in denen das KTS mittels Symptomen durch Selbstangaben bestimmt wurde, ohne den Nachweis eines Nervenleitgeschwindigkeitstests (NLG). Darüber hinaus fanden kaum biomechanische Expositionsmessungen beziehungsweise Beobachtungen statt. Die Exposition gegenüber biomechanischen Tätigkeiten wurde ausschließlich über Selbstangaben erfasst. Diese Beobachtung bestätigt ein kürzlich veröffentlichtes systematisches Review, das arbeitsbezogene MSE der oberen Extremitäten bei Gesundheitspersonal analysierte (Occhionero et al. 2014). Die Autoren schlussfolgern, dass eine biomechanische Expositionsanalyse für diese Berufsgruppe aus Mangel an Studien derzeit nicht möglich sei. Sie stellten jedoch fest, dass für bestimmte Berufsgruppen innerhalb des Gesundheitssektors höhere KTS-Prävalenzen angegeben werden: Dentalhygieniker (Symptome: 7–42%; Symptome und NLG: 6–8%), Zahnärzte (Symptome: 28%; Symptome und NLG: 5–16%), Sonographie- (Anamnese: 2–5%), Endoskopie- (Anamnese: 6%) und Anästhesiepersonal (Anamnese: 16%) (Occhionero et al. 2014). Repetitive Bewegungen in Kombination mit einem Fingerspitzengriff sowie dauerhafte Flexion der Handgelenke werden als typische Risikofaktoren für KTS bei Beschäftigten in der Zahnheilkunde oder Diagnostik diskutiert (Anton et al. 2002; Yamalik 2007).

Wie bereits erwähnt, war die epidemiologische Datenlage für Beschäftigte in Gesundheits- und Pflegeberufen spärlich. In den vergangenen Jahren wurden hingegen mehrere berufsübergreifende systematische Reviews (SRs) und Meta-Analysen zur Ätiologie von KTS publiziert. Also verfolgte diese Literaturstudie einen relativ neuen methodischen Ansatz, indem zunächst alle SRs und anschließend aktuelle Primärstudien systematisch erfasst, bewertet und analysiert wurden. Nach Cochrane wird diese Form der Evidenzsynthese aus mehreren SRs als „Overview of Systematic Reviews[3]" bezeichnet (Becker & Oxman 2008). Overviews geben einen breiten Überblick über die empirische Forschung zu einem bestimmten Thema (Cooper & Koenka 2012). Da SRs bereits innerhalb kürzester Zeit überholt sein können, wird empfohlen auch jüngste Veröffentlichungen zu berücksichtigen (Pieper et al. 2014; Whitlock et al. 2008).

Das Bundesministerium für Arbeit und Soziales hat 2009 auf Empfehlung des ärztlichen Sachverständigenbeirats „Berufskrankheiten" erwägt, das KTS in die BK-Verordnung aufzunehmen[4]. Danach galt es nach § 9 Abs. 1 SGB VII zu prüfen, ob und unter welchen sozialpolitischen Überlegungen und epidemiologischen Erkenntnissen ein KTS in die BK-Liste aufgenommen werden kann (Hoehne-Hückstädt et al. 2014). Die wissenschaftliche Begründung für das berufsbedingte KTS basiert auf einer selektiven Literaturübersicht ohne eingehende Qualitätsüberprüfung und Evidenzbewertung der eingeschlossenen Studien (Giersiepen & Spallek 2011). Mit der vorliegenden Arbeit wurde nun ein systematischer Ansatz angewandt, um relevante Arbeiten zu identifizieren, ihre Qualität zu bewerten und daraus evidenzbasierte Empfehlungen abzuleiten. Folglich ist dieses Overview eine Ergänzung zur wissenschaftlichen Begründung. Außerdem wird die neue Methode der Evidenzzusammenfassung und -bewertung kritisch diskutiert.

2.1.4 Belastende Körperhaltungen in der Altenpflege

Wenn von Wirbelsäulenbelastungen in der Pflege gesprochen wird, dann sind damit häufig Transfers und manuelle Handhabungen von Pflegebedürftigen gemeint (Yassi & Lockhart 2013). Pflegekräfte führen jedoch weitere Tätigkeiten aus,

---

[3] Weitere Synonyme: systematic review of systematic reviews; metareview; umbrella review; umbrella systematic review

[4] Definition der Berufskrankheit: „Druckschädigung des Nervus medianus im Karpaltunnel durch repetitive manuelle Tätigkeiten mit Beugung und Streckung der Handgelenke durch erhöhten Kraftaufwand der Hände oder durch Hand-Arm-Schwingungen".

die den Rücken ebenfalls erheblich beanspruchen können. Hodder et al. (2010) beobachteten, dass Pflegekräfte 50% ihrer Arbeitszeit mit Tätigkeiten wie Waschen, Pflegen, Anziehen, Essen reichen oder Betten machen verbringen. Lediglich 4% der Zeit wird für Transfers und Hebevorgänge gebraucht. Zu ähnlichen Ergebnissen kommen auch zwei weitere Beobachtungsstudien (Fiedler et al. 2012; Freitag et al. 2007). Bei Transfer- und Hebevorgängen werden zwar hohe Spitzenlasten beobachtet, diese Tätigkeiten sind aber lediglich für 10% der kumulativen lumbalen Bandscheiben-Druckkraft verantwortlich. Basispflegetätigkeiten und Sonstiges (z. B. Betten machen) machen dagegen 80% dieser Druckkraft aus (Holmes et al. 2010). Die Ausführung dieser Tätigkeiten erfordert ein häufiges Beugen oder Verdrehen des Oberkörpers sowie das Arbeiten in statischen Haltungen. Sagittale Neigungen über 60° (DIN 2002; ISO 2000) (Abbildung 6) wurden am häufigsten beim Betten machen (22%), Aufräumen (16%) und bei Basispflegetätigkeiten (16%) beobachtet (Freitag et al. 2007). Diese ungünstigen Körperhaltungen werden als zusätzliche Risikofaktoren für Rückenerkrankungen und -beschwerden diskutiert, da sie hohe Kraftanstrengung und Muskelkraft zur Bewältigung einer Aufgabe erfordern (OSHA 2009).

Interventionen zur Reduktion oder Prävention von körperlichen Belastungen und Rückenbeschwerden in der Pflege sind seit vielen Jahren Gegenstand der Forschung. Hauptsächlich wurde der Fokus auf Interventionen zur manuellen ergonomischen Handhabungen von Patienten gelegt (Best 1997; Videman et al. 1989), gefolgt von Maßnahmen zu körperlichen Betätigungen und Rückentrainings (Dehlin et al. 1981; Gundewall et al. 1993), Stressbewältigungsprogrammen (Horneij et al. 2001) sowie multifaktoriellen Strategien (Alexandre et al. 2001; Garg & Owen 1992). Vier systematische Reviews untersuchten den Effekt von Interventionen auf die Reduktion oder Verhinderung von Rückenbeschwerden und -verletzungen in der Pflege; sie kommen zu dem Schluss, dass Interventionen, die den Fokus ausschließlich auf manuelle Handhabung von Patienten legen, eine hohe Evidenz auf einen nicht vorhandenen Effekt zeigen. Hingegen weisen multifaktorielle Interventionen eine moderate Evidenz für eine Reduktion von Rückenbeschwerden auf (Bos et al. 2006; Dawson et al. 2007; Hignett 2003; Tullar et al. 2010). Da isoliert durchgeführte Interventionen zur manuellen Handhabung am Patienten keinen gewünschten Effekt erzielen, sollten andere arbeitsbezogene Faktoren zusätzlich in Betracht gezogen werden. Nach unserem Kenntnisstand wurden nur wenige Interventionsstudien durchgeführt, die den Effekt von ergonomischen Maßnahmen auf Körperhaltungen in der Pflege untersuchten (Engels et al. 1998; Fanello et al. 1999; Nussbaum & Torres 2001; Pohjonen et al. 1998). Sie beobachteten gegenüber Kontrollen einen signifikanten Anstieg von aufrechten und sicheren Körperhaltungen und eine Reduktion von ergonomischen Fehlern während der Arbeit.

Aus Vorstudien mit dem personengebundenen CUELA-Messsystem (Computer-unterstützte Erfassung und Langzeitanalyse von Muskel-Skelett-Belastungen) ist bekannt, dass ungünstige Körperhaltungen in der Pflege häufig vorkommen: Altenpflegekräfte arbeiteten im Vergleich zu Gesundheits- und Krankenpflegepersonal während einer Arbeitsschicht signifikant häufiger (112 versus 63 Minuten) in ungünstigen Neigungen über 20°; je intensiver die Pflegebedürftigkeit, umso häufiger und länger waren die ungünstigen Neigungen (Freitag et al. 2012). In einer Laborstudie wurde außerdem gezeigt, dass das Höherstellen der Betten und die Verwendung eines Hockers im Bad (pflegen im Sitzen) nicht nur zu einer Reduktion der ungünstigen Körperhaltungen führten, sondern die Probanden bei Einhaltung dieser ergonomischen Prinzipien die Tätigkeiten auch als weniger belastend empfanden (Freitag et al. 2014). Um die Pflegekräfte auf die häufig verkannten Risikofaktoren aufmerksam zu machen und sie dafür im Arbeitsalltag zu sensibilisieren, wurde ein praxisorientiertes Basisseminar zur Reduktion von ungünstigen Körperhaltungen entwickelt und in einer ersten Pilotstudie mit dem CUELA-Messsystem evaluiert.

2.2 Fragestellungen und Studienziele

2.2.1 Empirische Studie – Muskel-Skelett-Beschwerden bei Veterinären in Deutschland

Das Ziel der Studie war es, die MSB-Prävalenz und die daraus resultierenden körperlichen Einschränkungen sowie die Häufigkeit von Verletzungen im Bereich der distalen oberen Extremitäten und HWS bei praktizierenden Veterinären zu untersuchen und damit zusammenhängende Faktoren zu identifizieren. Dabei sollten folgende Fragen beantwortet werden:

1. *Wie hoch ist die 12-Monats-Prävalenz von MSB der oberen Extremitäten und HWS?*
2. *Wie häufig resultieren daraus körperliche Einschränkungen, die die Betroffenen bei der Ausführung ihrer Arbeit und in der Freizeit behindern?*
3. *Geben Großtierpraktiker häufiger Beschwerden im Bereich der oberen Extremitäten und HWS an als Veterinäre aus Klein- beziehungsweise Gemischttierpraxen?*
4. *Wie häufig kommen Unfälle vor, die zu Verletzungen im Bereich der oberen Extremitäten und HWS führen, und wie häufig werden diese durch Tiere verursacht?*
5. *Welche berufsbedingten und individuellen Faktoren stehen mit den funktionellen körperlichen Einschränkungen in den oberen Extremitäten und HWS im Zusammenhang?*

2.2.2 Empirische Studie – Gesundheitszustand, -verhalten und Perspektiven von Auszubildenden in pflegerischen und sozialen Berufen

Das Ziel der Studie war es, den Gesundheitszustand, das Gesundheitsverhalten sowie die Zukunftsperspektiven von Auszubildenden in Altenpflege, Gesundheits- und Krankenpflege (GuK) sowie Erziehung und sozialpädagogischer Assistenz (SPA) zu untersuchen und vergleichend darzustellen. Dabei sollten auch assoziierende Faktoren für den körperlichen und psychischen Gesundheitszustand der Auszubildenden ermittelt werden. Folgende Fragestellungen sollten beantwortet werden:

1. *Inwiefern unterscheiden sich die Auszubildenden in der Altenpflege, GuK sowie Erziehung und SPA hinsichtlich folgender Aspekte voneinander:*

   a. Gesundheitsverhalten (körperliche Aktivität, Ernährungsverhalten sowie Tabak- und Alkoholkonsum),

   b. Gesundheitszustand (Krankheiten und Beschwerden in den vorange-gangenen zwölf Monaten, Irritation und Selbstwirksamkeitserwartung),

   c. Arbeitssituation/Zukunftsperspektiven (Arbeitszufriedenheit, Intention den Beruf für weitere fünf Jahre auszuüben, Arbeitsbelastungen)?

2. *Welche gesundheitsbezogenen Faktoren stehen mit Muskel-Skelett-Erkrankungen sowie psychischen Beeinträchtigungen im Zusammenhang?*

2.2.3 Systematisches Overview über systematische Reviews und eine Meta-Analyse – berufsbedingtes KTS

Mit der systematischen Literaturarbeit sollte die bestehende Evidenz hinsichtlich des Zusammenhangs zwischen arbeitsbezogenen biomechanischen Belastungsfaktoren und KTS untersucht werden. Darüber hinaus sollte die Dosis-Wirkung-Beziehung der Expositionsfaktoren bestimmt werden. Folgende übergeordnete PEO-Fragestellung sollte beantwortet werden:

Besteht bei der Erwerbsbevölkerung (Population) ein Zusammenhang zwischen arbeitsbezogenen biomechanischen Belastungsfaktoren (Exposition) und KTS (Outcome)?

2.2.4 Evaluationsstudie – belastende Körperhaltungen in der Alten-pflege reduzieren

Im Rahmen der Evaluationsstudie wurde die Wirksamkeit eines Basisseminars zur Reduzierung von ungünstigen Körperhaltungen bei Altenpflegekräften messtechnisch evaluiert und auf die Umsetzbarkeit hin überprüft. Folgende Fragestellung wurde dabei untersucht:

Um welchen Anteil lassen sich ungünstige Körperhaltungen (Neigungswinkel über 20° beziehungsweise über 60°) nach der Umsetzung der ergonomischen Maßnahme reduzieren und wie effektiv ist diese Maßnahme?

2.3   Material und Methodik

2.3.1 Empirische Studie – Muskel-Skelett-Beschwerden bei Veterinären in Deutschland

Zur Erfassung von Häufigkeit und Schwere der MSB wurde 2011 ein Survey unter den Mitgliedern der Landestierärztekammern Baden-Württemberg, Bayern, Berlin, Brandenburg, Niedersachsen, Schleswig-Holstein und Westfalen-Lippe durchgeführt. Insgesamt nahmen 3.174 Tierärzte an der Befragung teil (Rücklaufquote: 38,4%). Dazu wurde der standardisierte Nordic Questionnaire verwendet (Kuorinka et al. 1987). Mit diesem Instrument werden Symptome wie Stechen, Schmerzen, Missempfindungen oder Bewegungseinschränkungen in den vorausgegangenen zwölf Monaten erfragt. Es wurden Fragen zur Dauer der Beschwerden, zu Einschränkungen der allgemeinen Aktivitäten und beruflichen Tätigkeiten gestellt. Zusätzlich wurde erfragt, ob die Beschwerden durch berufsbedingte Unfälle verursacht worden seien. Diese Unfälle wurden danach differenziert, ob sie im Zusammenhang mit Tieren oder Verrichtungen während der Arbeitszeit entstanden sind (z. B. Stürze oder Wegeunfälle). Neben soziodemografischen und berufsbezogenen Variablen (z. B. Praxisart) wurden die Teilnehmer um Einschätzung zur Häufigkeit der von ihnen jährlich durchgeführten tierärztlichen Tätigkeiten gebeten, z. B. Geburtshilfe, rektale/vaginale Untersuchungen (Scuffham et al. 2010b). Skalen, die quantitative Arbeitsbelastungen und „personal burnout" erfassen, wurden aus der deutschen Version des Copenhagen Psychosocial Questionnaire (COPSOQ) entnommen (Nübling et al. 2005). Unterschiede in den kategorialen Variablen wurden mit dem Pearson-Chi-Quadrat-Test analysiert. Zunächst wurden die Daten mittels univariater Methoden untersucht. Um die Wahrscheinlichkeit von Typ-I-Fehlern zu verringern, wurde der Alpha-Wert auf $p < 0,01$ gesetzt. Variablen, die MSB signifikant in der jeweiligen Körperregion beeinflussten, wurden für die multivariate Modellbildung gewählt; diese erfolgte schrittweise rückwärts unter Verwendung des Change-Kriteriums.

2.3.2 Empirische Studie – Gesundheitszustand, -verhalten und Perspektiven von Auszubildenden in pflegerischen und sozialen Berufen

Auszubildende zum Altenpfleger, GuK, Erzieher sowie SPA wurden hinsichtlich ihres Gesundheitszustandes, -verhaltens und ihrer Zukunftsperspektiven befragt Diese Querschnittsstudie fand zwischen Januar und März 2014 an Hamburger

Berufsschulen statt. Insgesamt wurden 16 von 20 Berufsschulen dieser Fachrichtungen kontaktiert und um Teilnahme gebeten; acht Schulen sicherten ihre Teilnahme an der Befragung zu. Aus Verfügbarkeitsgründen übernahmen die Schulleitungen die Zuweisungen der zu befragenden Schulklassen und Jahrgänge. Zu diesem Zeitpunkt wurden alle Jahrgänge und Altersklassen in das Studienkollektiv eingeschlossen. Die Befragung fand in den Unterrichtsstunden statt.

Insgesamt beteiligten sich 402 Auszubildende an der Befragung (Rücklaufquote: 99%). Das Alter der Teilnehmenden variierte erheblich (16 bis 52 Jahre). Jüngere zeigten gegenüber älteren Befragten (>30 Jahre) einen deutlich riskanteren Alkoholkonsum und ein ungünstigeres Ernährungsverhalten. Folglich wurden nur Auszubildende zwischen dem 16. und 30. Lebensjahr in die endgültige Analyse eingeschlossen (n=354; 88%). Ein Cut-off von 30 Jahren wurde unter anderem gewählt, um die vorliegenden Ergebnisse mit der Altersgruppe der 18- bis 29-Jährigen aus der Studie zur Gesundheit Erwachsener in Deutschland (DEGS1) vergleichen zu können. Das Erhebungsinstrument setzte sich aus bereits validierten und erprobten Skalen und Items zusammen, die zum Teil an die Zielgruppe angepasst wurden (Abbildung 3; Referenzen siehe Publikation 2).

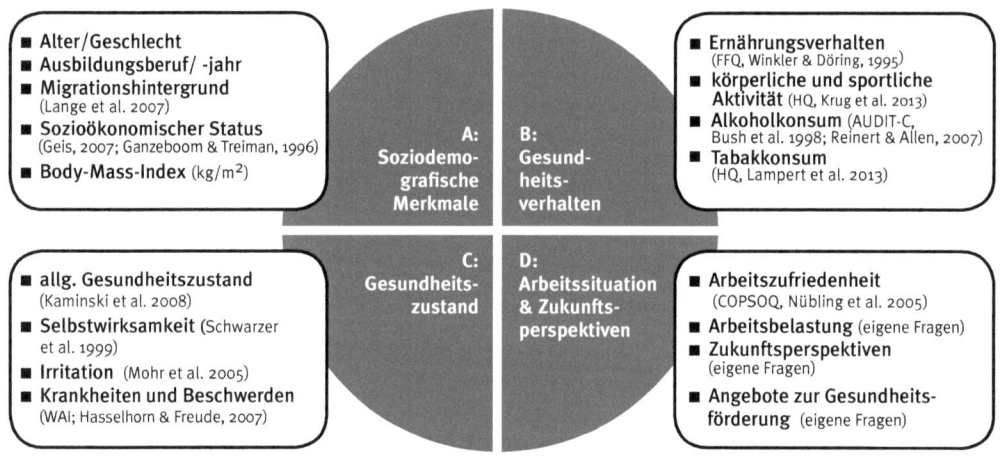

Abbildung 3: Zusammensetzung des Fragebogens bei Auszubildenden

Unterschiede zwischen den Ausbildungsberufen wurden für die kategorialen Variablen mit dem Pearson-Chi-Quadrat-Test ermittelt. Bei Mittelwertvergleichen wurden sowohl einfaktorielle Varianzanalysen (ANOVA und Scheffé-Post-hoc-

Tests) als auch nicht parametrische Testverfahren (Kruskal-Wallis-H-Test) verwendet. Mittels logistischen Regressionsanalysen wurden gesundheitsbezogene Faktoren auf ihren Zusammenhang mit MSE und psychischen Beeinträchtigungen untersucht. Es wurden hierarchische Modelle gebildet; im ersten Schritt wurden Variablen aus univariaten Analysen eingeschlossen (p <0,05) und im zweiten Schritt wurden weitere Variablen mit einem Signifikanzniveau von p <0,25 hinzugefügt, sofern diese zu einer wesentlichen Modellverbesserung beitrugen.

2.3.3 Systematisches Overview über systematische Reviews und eine Meta-Analyse – berufsbedingtes KTS

Die Literatursuche und -analyse fand in zwei Schritten statt. Im ersten Schritt wurden systematische Reviews (SRs) und im zweiten Schritt Primärstudien identifiziert. Das Vorgehen orientierte sich jeweils an dem Methodenpapier von PEROSH[5] (2012) und der MOOSE-Checkliste[6] (Stroup et al. 2000). Eine elektronische Literatursuche wurde in den Datenbanken MEDLINE, EMBASE, CINAHL und COCHRANE durchgeführt. Der eingeschlossene Publikationszeitraum für SRs beschränkte sich auf 1998 bis 2014 und für aktuelle Primärstudien auf 2011 bis 2014. Zur Identifizierung ätiologischer Studien im beruflichen Kontext wurde ein sensitiver Suchstring von Mattioli et al. (2010) in Kombination mit den Begriffen für Exposition, Outcome und Studiendesign verwendet. Sechs Sprachen wurden berücksichtigt[7]. Die Studien wurden von zwei Reviewern unabhängig voneinander ausgewählt und bewertet. Folgende Einschlussfaktoren wurden berücksichtigt: (a) Erwerbstätige, (b) mindestens ein biomechanischer Faktor, (c) KTS als primäres Outcome und nicht als Begleiterkrankung, (d) SRs und Meta-Analysen. Bei Primärstudien wurden außerdem nur Studien eingeschlossen, die eine konservative KTS-Definition[8] verwendeten.

Der wiederholte Einschluss von Primärstudien in mehr als nur einem SR zur selben Fragestellung kann die Ergebnisse verzerren. Bei der Durchführung von

---

[5] PEROSH — Partnership for European Research in Occupational Safety and Health, Working Group Clearinghouse of Systematic Reviews

[6] MOOSE – Meta-analysis of Observational Studies in Epidemiology

[7] Sprachen: Deutsch, Englisch, Italienisch, Spanisch, Portugiesisch und Russisch

[8] KTS Definition: (a) Ein positiver Befund des Nervenleitgeschwindigkeitstests (z. B. Dysfunktion des N. medianus) und (b) entweder ein positiver klinischer Befund (Phalen's- oder Tinel's-Test) oder Symptome wie Parästhesien, Taubheitsgefühle oder Schmerzen (Barcenilla et al. 2012)

Overviews sollte daher der Überschneidungsgrad von Primärstudien zwischen den SRs bestimmt werden. Um dem Rechnung zu tragen, wurde die „Corrected Covered Area" (CCA) nach der Methode von Pieper et al. (2014) ermittelt. CCA[9] kann interpretiert werden als die Überschneidungsfläche von Studien, die mindestens zweimal in SRs erscheinen, nach Bereinigung aller Primärstudien bei ihrer ersten Zählung (siehe Formel 1).

$$CCA = \frac{(N-r)}{(rc-r)}$$

Formel 1: Covered Corrected Area: N ist die Anzahl der eingeschlossenen Publikationen (u. a. Doppelzählungen) in der Evidenzsynthese einzelner SRs; r ist die Anzahl der Index-Publikationen (einzelne Primärstudien) und c die Anzahl der SRs.

Die Bewertung der methodischen Qualität von SRs wurde mit dem AMSTAR-R-Instrument[10] (maximal 44 Punkte) vorgenommen (Kung et al. 2010). Die Beurteilung von Primärstudien fand in Anlehnung an die Qualitätskriterien von van Rijn et al. (2009) und Ariens et al. (2001) statt. Diese wurden an die eigene Fragestellung angepasst und zum Summenscore (maximal 20 Punkte) zusammengefasst.

Die Qualität der Evidenz wurde nach einem qualitativen Ansatz separat nach Art der beruflichen Exposition bestimmt. Dabei wurde die methodische Validität der SRs (AMSTAR-R-Score) und die Konsistenz der Ergebnisse (Effektrichtung und Signifikanz) zwischen den SRs berücksichtigt (Walton et al. 2013). Die Ergebnisse der Primärstudien dienten unterstützend zur Abschätzung der Qualität der Evidenz, indem sowohl ihre methodische Validität als auch die Konsistenz berücksichtigt wurden, z. B. wenn mindestens zwei valide Primärstudien ($\geq$14 Punkte) konsistente Ergebnisse aufwiesen, wurde die Qualität der Evidenz aus den SRs heraufgestuft. Vergleichbare aktuelle Primärstudien wurden miteinander gepoolt und mittels Forest Plots dargestellt. Als Effektschätzer wurde das relative Risiko (RR) berechnet. Die Heterogenität wurde mit dem Chi-Quadrat (χ^2) untersucht (p <0,10). Der I^2-Test wurde verwendet, um Unterschiede zwischen den Studien zu quantifizieren. Bei Vorliegen von Heterogenität (χ^2, p-Wert <0,10 und I^2 >50%) wurde das Random-Effect-Modell verwendet (Deeks et al. 2008).

---

[9] CCA-Werte zwischen 0 und 5 deuten auf einen leichten, zwischen 6 und 10 auf einen moderaten, zwischen 11 und 15 auf einen hohen und Werte über 15 auf einen sehr hohen Überschneidungsgrad hin.

[10] AMSTAR – Assessment of Multiple Systematic Reviews – Revised

2.3.4 Evaluationsstudie – belastende Körperhaltungen in der Altenpflege reduzieren

Zur Reduzierung von ungünstigen Körperhaltungen wurden ein zweitägiges Basisseminar und zwei halbtägige Nachschulungen als beratende Begleitung während des Frühdienstes für die Probanden konzipiert. Die Evaluation dieser Intervention erfolgte mit dem personengebundenen CUELA-Messsystem (Ellegast et al. 2009), Videoanalysen und fragebogenbasierter Befragung. Abbildung 4 zeigt den Ablauf des Schulungskonzeptes und die Zeitpunkte der messtechnischen beziehungsweise telefonischen Evaluation.

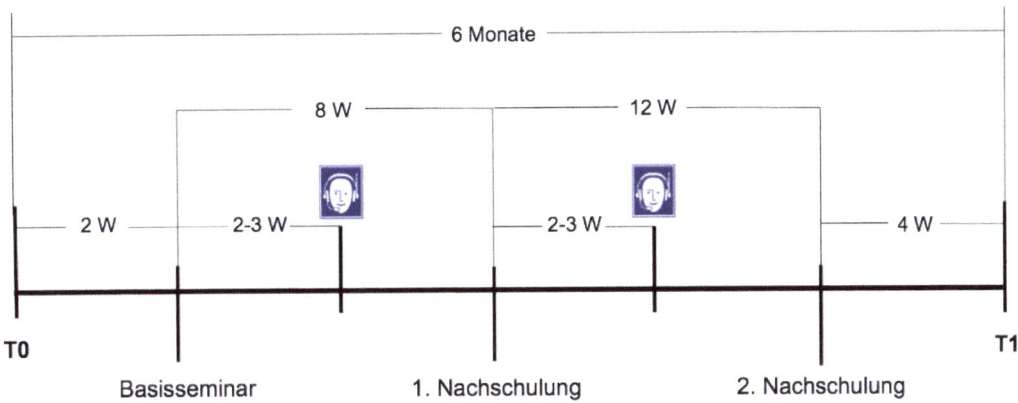

Abbildung 4 Ablauf des Schulungskonzeptes und Evaluation

Sensoren an der Brust- und Lendenwirbelsäule ermöglichen eine dreidimensionale Darstellung der Oberkörperneigungen. Dadurch war eine realitätsgetreue kinematische Rekonstruktion der Bewegungen von Probanden möglich. Zu jeder Messung wurden die Probanden mit einer Videokamera über die gesamte Schicht begleitet. Mithilfe einer speziell entwickelten Software (WIDAAN 2.79) wurden die Messdaten und Videoaufnahmen synchronisiert. Alle eingenommenen Körperhaltungen und Bewegungen eines Probanden wurden entsprechend der durchgeführten Tätigkeit zugeordnet (Abbildung 5).

Um eine Bewertung von Arbeitshaltungen und ihres möglichen Schädigungspotenzials auf den Bewegungsapparat zu untersuchen, wurden Abweichungen der Gelenkwinkel von der Neutralstellung betrachtet. Sagittale Neigungen zwischen 0° und 20° wurden nach ISO 11226 (ISO 2000) und DIN EN 1005-4 (DIN 2005) dem akzeptablen Bereich zugeordnet und entsprachen einer aufrechten Körperhaltung. In dieser Position ist der Druck auf die Bandscheibe am geringsten. Er steigt mit

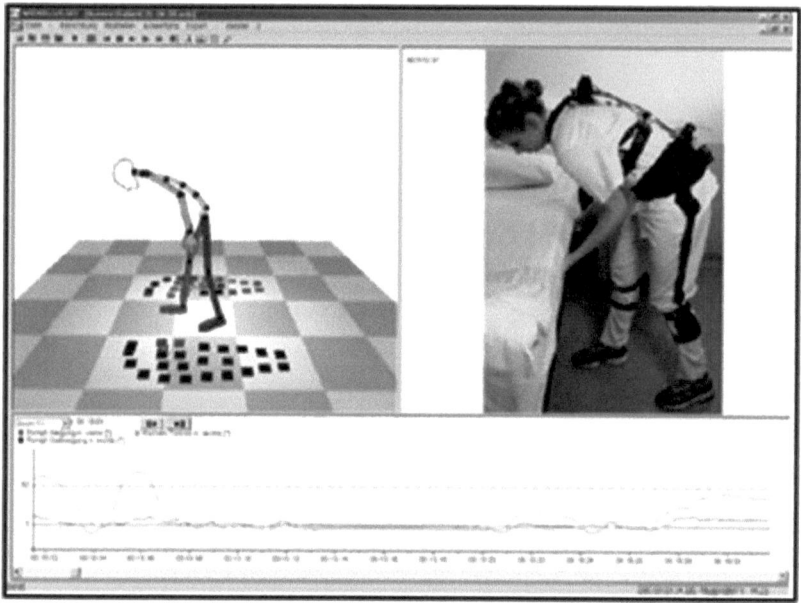

Abbildung 5 Benutzeroberfläche der WIDAAN-Software zur Evaluation der Messdaten

zunehmendem Grad der sagittalen Neigung (Wilke et al. 1999). Sagittale Neigungen zwischen 20° und 60° wurden als bedingt akzeptabel und über 60° als nicht akzeptabel eingestuft (DIN 2005; ISO 2000) (Abbildung 6). Es wurde die Häufigkeit der sagittalen Neigungen ($\geq$20°, $\geq$60°) gemessen sowie der Zeitanteil an der gesamten Arbeitsschicht ermittelt.

Wenn Probanden in einer sagittalen Neigung länger als vier Sekunden verharrten, wurde diese als statisch definiert (DIN EN 1005-1, 2002). Die Funktionsweise des Messsystems sowie die ergonomische Bewertung der Körperhaltungen in der Alten- und Krankenpflege wurden in früheren Veröffentlichungen ausführlich beschrieben (Freitag et al. 2007; 2012).

Da die Pflegeintensität einzelner Bewohner und somit auch die erforderliche Grundpflege erheblich variieren, wurde in einer Vorstudie ein Basis-Pflegeintensitätsscore entwickelt (Freitag et al. 2012). Mittels Videoanalysen wurden individuelle Basis-Pflegetätigkeiten identifiziert (z. B. Betten machen, waschen, rasieren, anziehen etc.) und nach Pflegeintensität der Bewohner der entsprechenden Schicht und Pflegekraft zugeordnet. Je höher der Gesamtscore, umso höher war die Pflegeintensität (Freitag et al. 2012). Dieser Score wurde für beide Zeitpunkte erfasst, um die Variabilität der Pflegeintensität zu berücksichtigen.

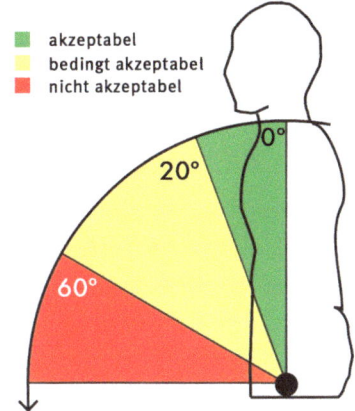

akzeptabel
bedingt akzeptabel
nicht akzeptabel

0°
20°
60°

Abbildung 6 Winkelstellungen des Oberkörpers nach DIN EN 1005-4, ISO 11226

Das Basisseminar wurde entwickelt, um Pflegekräfte für die häufigen körperlichen Anstrengungen im Pflegealltag zu sensibilisieren. Es bestand zu gleichen Teilen aus Theorie zu Körperhaltungen in der Pflege, Körperwahrnehmung und Entspannung sowie der praktischen Umsetzung am Pflegebett und im Badezimmer. Jede Pflegekraft sollte die Basis-Pflegetätigkeiten am Bewohnerbett (Abbildung 7) sowie im Bad (Abbildung 8) zweimal direkt hintereinander bei zwei Betthöhen (Oberschenkel- und hüfthoch) beziehungsweise mit und ohne Hocker durchführen. Durch diesen direkten Vergleich sollten sie feststellen, wie entlastend das Arbeiten am hochgestellten Bett beziehungsweise sitzend auf einem Hocker ist. Außerdem wurden in diesem Seminar ergonomische Hilfsmittel wie Pflegekörbchen und Wäschewanne vorgestellt. Damit sollten mehrmalige sagittale Neigungen zum Nachtschrank/Boden verhindert werden (Abbildung 9).

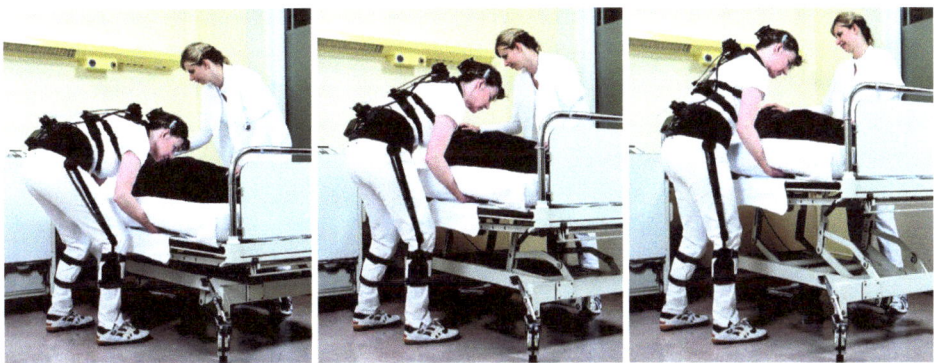

Abbildung 7 Basis-Pflegetätigkeiten am Bewohnerbett bei drei unterschiedlichen Betthöhen

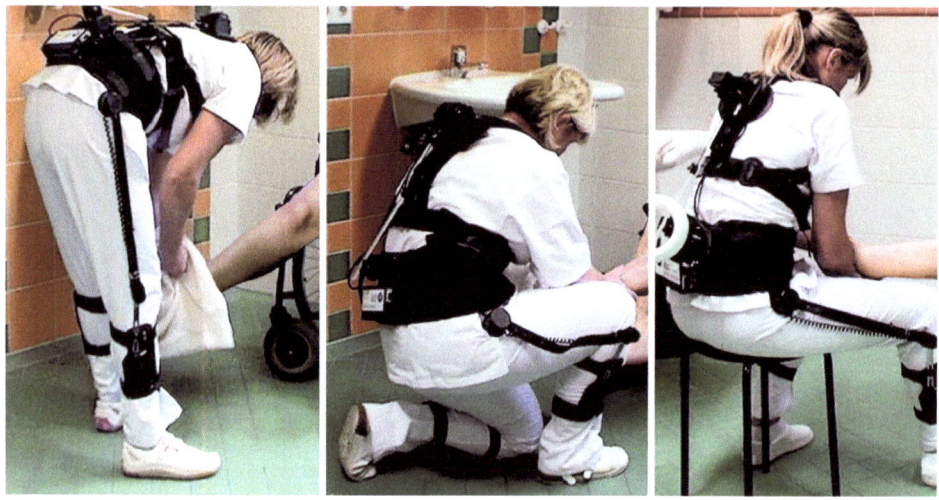

Abbildung 8 Basis-Pflegetätigkeiten im Bad in stehender, hockender und sitzender Position

| Ergonomisches Bewohnerzimmer | Einsatz eines Pflegekörbchens | Einsatz einer Wäschewanne |

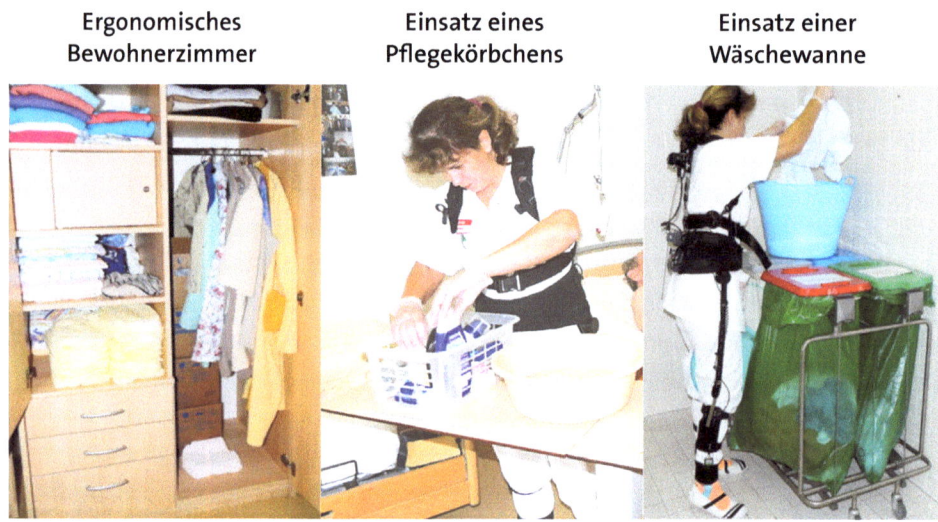

Abbildung 9 Ergonomische Umgestaltung und Hilfsmittel

Unterschiede zwischen zwei Messzeitpunkten wurden mittels T-Test beziehungsweise als nicht parametrische Alternative mit dem Wilcoxon-Test bei verbundenen Stichproben ermittelt. Dabei wurden die Mediane, Interquartilsabstand sowie nicht parametrische Hodges-Lehman-Schätzer mit 95%-Konfidenzintervall (KI) angegeben. Zusätzlich wurden die relative Veränderung zwischen den zwei Zeitpunkten mithilfe dieser Gleichung bestimmt: $((T1-T0)/T0)*100$. Zweiseitige P-Werte $<0{,}05$ wurden als statistisch signifikant betrachtet. Die Analysen wurden mit IBM SPSS Version 22.0 durchgeführt.

2.4 Ergebnisse

2.4.1 Empirische Studie – Muskel-Skelett-Beschwerden bei Veterinären in Deutschland

Die 12-Monats-Prävalenz von MSB zeigte je nach Körperregion erhebliche Unterschiede. Am häufigsten betroffen waren die HWS-Region und der Schulterbereich. Großtierpraktiker gaben signifikant häufiger MSB an den distalen oberen Extremitäten an als Klein- und Gemischttierpraktiker (Abbildung 10).

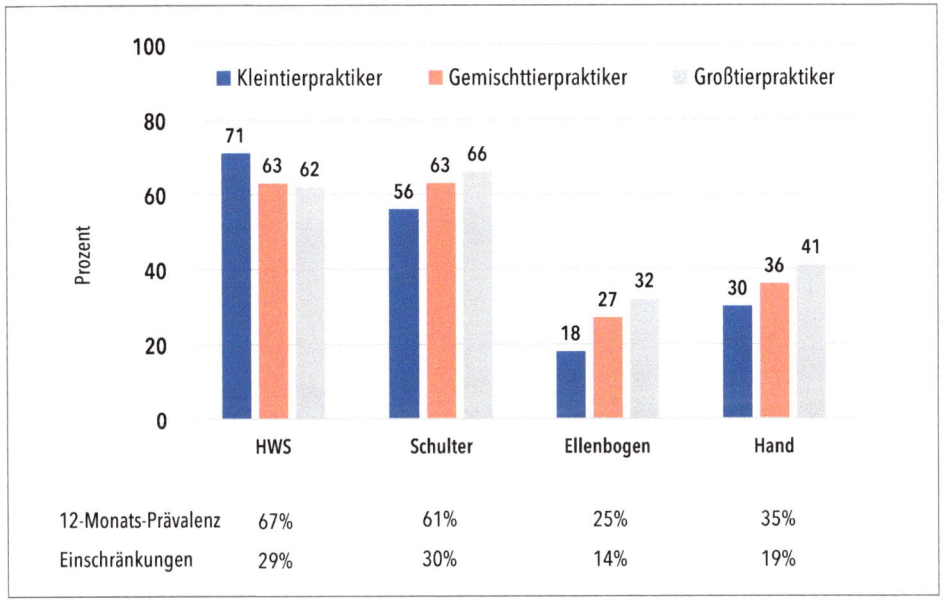

Abbildung 10 Zwölf-Monats-Prävalenzen von MSB, stratifiziert nach Praxisart

Beschwerden, die durch Arbeitsunfälle verursacht wurden, traten häufig im Bereich der Hand (14%) und der Schulter (11%) auf. Als Unfallursache an den distalen Extremitäten wurden vorwiegend Tiere genannt. Im Bereich der HWS waren andere Faktoren ursächlich (z. B. Schleudertrauma). Männliche Veterinäre gaben häufiger an, Verletzungen an der HWS (11% vs. 7%), den Schultern (23% vs. 10%), Ellenbogen (21 % vs. 13%) und der Hand (37% vs. 30%) zu erleiden als ihre weiblichen Kolleginnen. Die Unfallrate stieg mit dem Alter der Veterinäre. Bezogen auf die Praxisart zeigte sich, dass Groß- und Gemischttierpraktiker signifikant häufiger Unfälle (im Bereich der HWS, Schulter und Ellenbogen; Ausnahme: Hand) meldeten als Kleintierpraktiker (keine Tabelle).

MSB in den unterschiedlichen Körperregionen der oberen Extremitäten wurden getrennt analysiert; alle wesentlichen Ergebnisse aus den multivariaten Regressionsanalysen sind in der Abbildung 11 dargestellt. Je nach Körperregion trugen folgende demografische, arbeitsbedingte oder psychische Faktoren wesentlich zur Beschwerdelast bei: höheres Alter, Geschlecht, frühere Verletzungen, BMI, Praxistyp, häufig durchgeführte veterinäre Tätigkeiten wie zahnmedizinische Eingriffe, rektale Untersuchungen und Geburtshilfe sowie hohe Arbeitsanforderungen und erhöhte Burnout-Symptomatik.

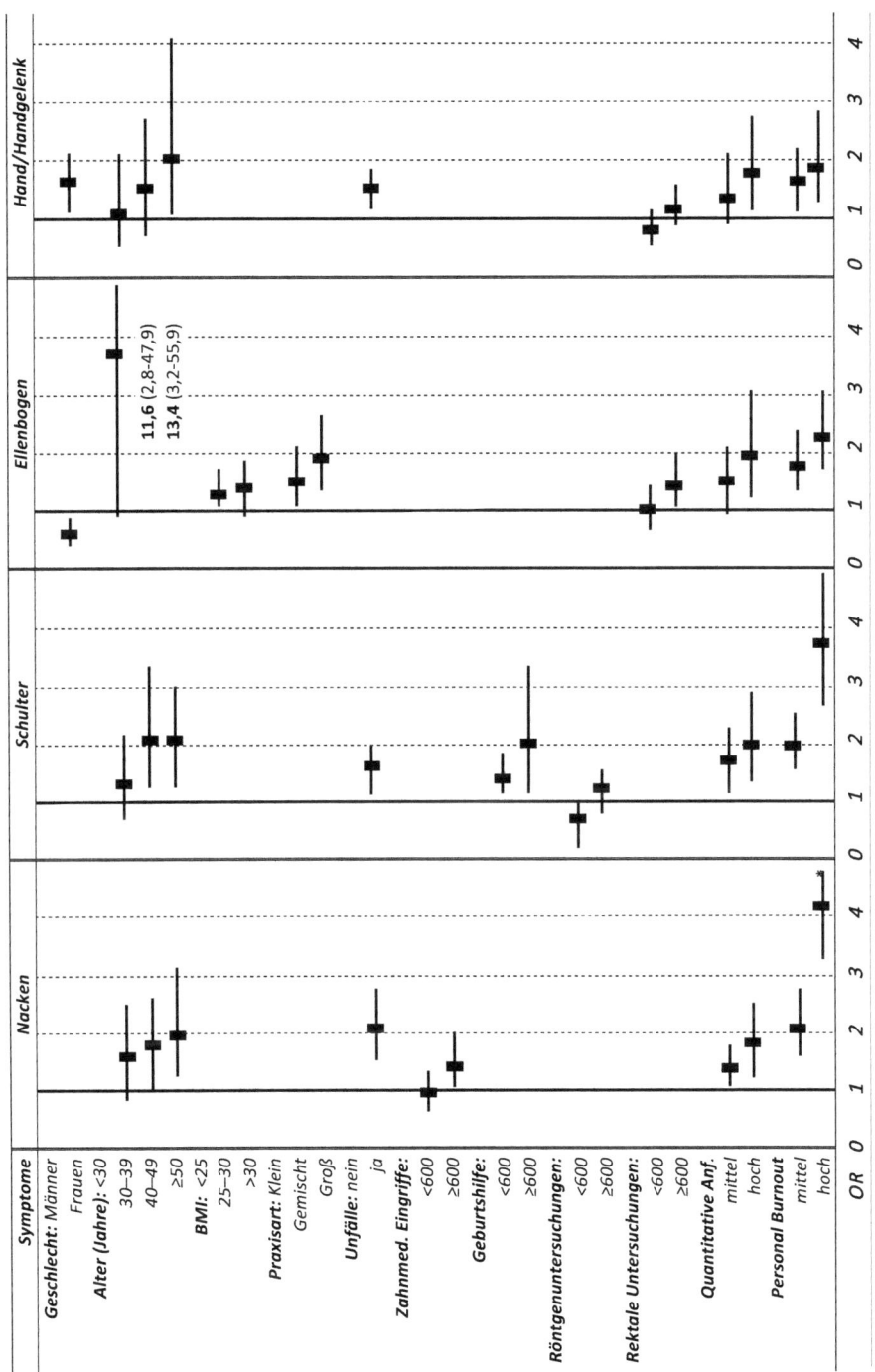

Anm.: *Erste Variablenzeile ist die Referenzkategorie (bei tierärztlichen Tätigkeiten und psychischer Belastung: „keine" beziehungsweise „gering").*

Abbildung 11 Einflussfaktoren für Funktionseinschränkungen, Endmodell: OR mit 95%-KI

2.4.2 Empirische Studie – Gesundheitsverhalten, -zustand und Perspektiven von Auszubildenden in pflegerischen und sozialen Berufen

Im Gegensatz zu Schülern in der GuK (15,5%) und Erziehung/SPA (22%) gab etwa ein Viertel der Altenpflegeschüler an, sich gar nicht sportlich zu betätigen. Ein ungünstiges Ernährungsverhalten wiesen die Auszubildenden in der Altenpflege (41%) und in der Erziehung/SPA (46%) auf. Bei GuK-Schülern waren es lediglich 28%. In allen Gruppen lag der Anteil der täglichen und gelegentlichen Raucher über 35%. In der Altenpflege war er mit 55% am höchsten. Riskanter Alkoholkonsum[11] lag bei allen Ausbildungsgruppen bei über 40%.

Die Mehrheit schätzte ihren allgemeinen Gesundheitszustand als gut oder sehr gut ein. Rund ein Drittel der Auszubildenden in der Altenpflege und Erziehung/SPA galten anhand ihres BMI als übergewichtig oder adipös. Bei GuK-Schülern lag der Anteil bei 22%. Bei der Auflistung von Krankheiten und Beschwerden in den vorangegangenen zwölf Monaten wurden psychische Beeinträchtigungen mit 38% und MSE mit 35% am häufigsten genannt. Als betroffene Körperregionen wurden in allen drei Gruppen am häufigsten der Rücken sowie die Knieregion angegeben. Ergebnisse aus dem multivariaten Modell zeigten, dass Auszubildende, die psychisch beansprucht (OR 1,8; 95%-KI 1,1–3,1) und zwischen 23 und 26 Jahre alt waren (OR 3,1; 95%-KI 1,4–6,7), eine erhöhte Wahrscheinlichkeit hatten, an MSE zu erkranken als nicht beanspruchte und unter 19-Jährige. Das Modell erzielte eine Varianzaufklärung von 18%. Irritation, Arbeitszufriedenheit und sozioökonomischer Status zeigten im multivariaten Modell keinen statistisch signifikanten Zusammenhang mit dem Zielkriterium.

Stratifiziert nach dem Lehrjahr war die Irritation bei den Auszubildenden im zweiten und dritten Lehrjahr signifikant höher (24,2; ± 10,5 beziehungsweise 24; ± 11,6) als im ersten Jahr (21,1; ± 9,4). Es gab jedoch keine statistisch relevanten Unterschiede zwischen den Ausbildungsberufen. Auszubildende in der Erziehung/SPA (68,2; ± 16,7) zeigten im Gegensatz zu Altenpflegeschülern (62,1; ± 15,9) und GuK (57,4; ± 15,2) die höchsten Arbeitszufriedenheitswerte an. Diese nahmen vom ersten (68,6; ± 13,8) bis zum dritten Lehrjahr (53,1; ± 16,9) signifikant ab. Häufig wur-

---

[11] Die Kurzform des „Alcohol Use Disorders Identification Tests" (AUDIT-C) beinhaltet drei Items. Pro Item werden 0–4 Punkte vergeben, sodass maximal 12 Punkte erreicht werden können. Ein riskanter Alkoholkonsum gilt bei Frauen ab drei und bei Männern ab vier Punkten (Reinert & Allen 2007).

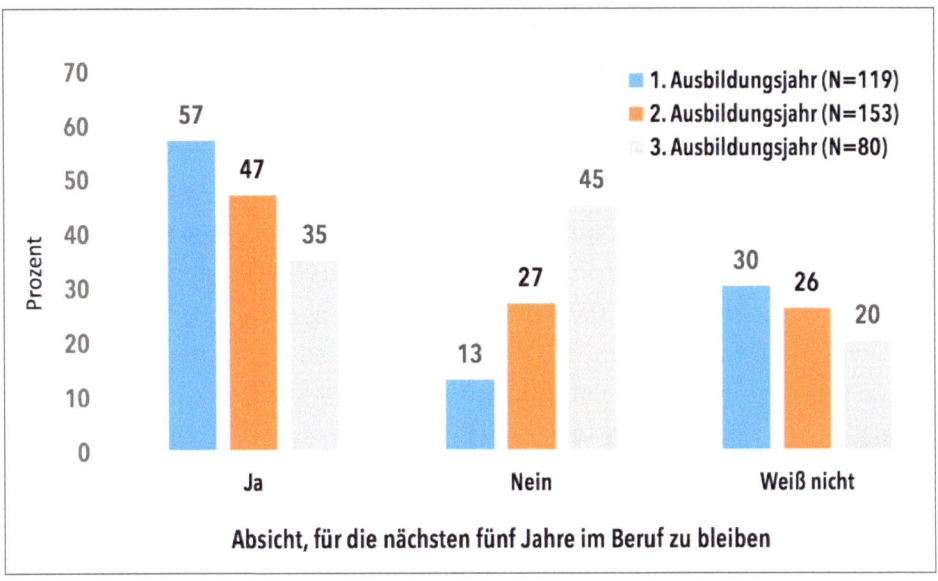

Abbildung 12 Wunsch zum Verbleib im Beruf, stratifiziert nach Ausbildungsjahr

den Zeitdruck, Stress, körperliche und psychische Anstrengung, Personalmangel, Arbeitszeiten sowie psychosoziale Anforderungen im Team als stark belastende Faktoren im Arbeitsalltag genannt. 62% der Auszubildenden in der Erziehung/SPA konnten sich vorstellen, den gelernten Beruf auch in den nächsten fünf Jahren auszuüben. In der Altenpflege waren es knapp die Hälfte und in der GuK lediglich 36%. Die Intention, in dem Beruf zu bleiben, nahm mit jedem Lehrjahr signifikant ab (Abbildung 12).

Auf die Frage nach den Wünschen für ihre Arbeitssituation, um in dem gelernten Beruf motiviert zu bleiben und ihn dauerhaft auszuüben, antworteten jeweils mehr als die Hälfte der Auszubildenden, dass sie sich eine bessere Bezahlung beziehungsweise ein besseres Ansehen in der Bevölkerung wünschten. Bei den Auszubildenden der Altenpflege und GuK wurde am zweithäufigsten der Wunsch nach mehr Personal geäußert (44% und 53%). In der Erziehung und SPA gaben 25% den Wunsch nach einem besseren Arbeitsklima im Team an.

2.4.3 Systematisches Overview über systematische Reviews und eine Meta-Analyse – berufsbedingtes KTS

Nach einem systematischen Auswahlverfahren wurden im ersten Schritt zehn systematische Reviews (SRs) in die Analyse eingeschlossen. Diese SRs berücksichtigten 143 Primärstudien, die bis zu 314-mal zitiert wurden. Im zweiten Schritt wurden sieben aktuelle Primärstudien in die Evidenzsynthese einbezogen; vier davon wurden in der Meta-Analyse zur Klärung der Dosis-Wirkung-Beziehung berücksichtigt. Alle vier Studien wiesen eine sehr gute Qualität auf und verwendeten den American Conference of Governmental Industrial Hygienists (ACGIH) Threshold Limit Value (TLV) für Hand Activity Level (HAL)[12]. Ein Wert unterhalb des Aktionslimits (AL <0,56) wird als unbedenklich, zwischen AL und dem Schwellenlimit (TLV) als bedenklich und oberhalb des TLV (>0,78) als gefährdend eingestuft. Der TLV sollte nicht überschritten werden; AL dient als Kontrollkategorie (ACGIH 2002). Alle hier zusammengefassten Ergebnisse können aus der Publikation 3 entnommen werden (SRs siehe Tabelle 3; Primärstudien siehe Tabelle 4).

Zwei qualitativ gute SRs stellten einen Zusammenhang zwischen **Repetition** und KTS fest. Weitere SRs von geringer Qualität lieferten keine widersprüchlichen Ergebnisse. Vier aktuelle Primärstudien von hoher Qualität bestätigten diesen Zusammenhang. Einer Primärstudie zufolge standen Berufe, die häufig repetitive Bewegungsabläufe erfordern, in einem signifikanten Zusammenhang mit KTS. Dies galt sowohl für eine kurze als auch für eine lange Beschäftigungsdauer (Evanoff et al. 2014). Gemäß den zuvor definierten Kriterien wurde die Qualität der Evidenz für einen positiven Zusammenhang zwischen Repetition und KTS als hoch eingestuft.

Zwei qualitativ gute SRs zeigten einen Zusammenhang zwischen **Kraftaufwand** und KTS. Weitere SRs von geringer Qualität lieferten keine widersprüchlichen Erkenntnisse. Vier Primärstudien von hoher Qualität kamen ebenfalls zu dem Ergebnis, dass Kraftaufwand in einem signifikanten Zusammenhang mit KTS steht. Die Längsschnittergebnisse belegen, dass Kraftanstrengungen, die mehr als 20% der Arbeitszeit ausmachten, das Risiko für KTS verdreifachten; ab 60% der Zeit

---

[12] Dieser Score ermittelt die durchschnittliche Aktivität (HAL) und Spitzenkraft (PF) der Hand durch Beobachtungen. HAL basiert auf der Bewegungshäufigkeit und dem Arbeitszyklus (Verhältnis von Aktivität und Erholungsphasen). PF basiert auf der max. Kraftanwendung während eines regulären Arbeitstaktes.

erhöhte sich das Risiko auf das 20-Fache. BMI fungierte als Confounder (Burt et al. 2013). Die Qualität der Evidenz wurde als hoch eingestuft.

Zwei Meta-Analysen untersuchten die Beziehung zwischen **kombinierten Belastungsmustern** an der Hand und KTS; sie stellten eine Verdopplung des Risikos fest, jedoch mit dem Nachweis einer signifikanten Heterogenität (Barcenilla et al. 2012; Spahn et al. 2012). Handbelastungen innerhalb der oberen ACGIH-TLV-Tertile gingen mit einer signifikant höheren KTS-Inzidenz und -Prävalenz einher (Spahn et al. 2012). Diese Ergebnisse konnten auch in der vorliegenden Meta-Analyse repliziert werden. Demnach zeigte die Analyse, dass bereits bei einem mittleren HAL für TLV das Risiko erhöht ist (RR: 1,5; 95%-KI 1,02–2,31; Abbildung 13). Bei der Überschreitung des TLV verdoppelt sich das Risiko für KTS (RR: 2,0; 95%-KI 1,46–2,82; Abbildung 14). Folglich wurde die Qualität der Evidenz für diese Beziehung als hoch eingestuft.

Zwei qualitativ gute SRs fanden einen Zusammenhang zwischen **Vibration** und KTS. Ihre Ergebnisse stützten die Autoren auf Studien mit Querschnitts- und Fall-Kontroll-Design (Barcenilla et al. 2012; van Rijn et al. 2009). Weitere SRs lieferten keine widersprüchlichen Erkenntnisse. Sie schlussfolgerten, dass Vibration zwar ein plausibler Faktor, jedoch die Evidenzlage für einen kausalen Zusammenhang unzureichend sei. In aktuellen Primärstudien von hoher Qualität stellte Vibration keinen unabhängigen, starken Prädiktor für KTS dar. Folglich wurde die Qualität der Evidenz als moderat eingestuft.

Es wurden in den Reviews inkonsistente Ergebnisse für den Zusammenhang zwischen **Flexion und Extension** des Handgelenks und KTS beobachtet. Mehrere Reviews berichten von einer signifikanten Heterogenität der eingeschlossenen Studien (Barcenilla et al. 2012; Spahn et al. 2012; You et al. 2014). Zwei aktuelle Primärstudien von hoher Qualität konnten keinen Nachweis für diese Beziehung liefern. Folglich wurde die Qualität der Evidenz hinsichtlich der Beziehung zwischen chronischer Flexions- und Extensionshaltung der Hand und KTS als gering eingestuft.

Eine Meta-Analyse von guter Qualität zeigte, dass die epidemiologische Evidenz hinsichtlich einer positiven Beziehung zwischen **PC-Arbeit** und KTS unzureichend ist (Mediouni et al. 2014). Weitere SRs bestätigen diese Erkenntnisse. In den aktuellen Primärstudien wird dieser Zusammenhang nicht untersucht. Gemäß den postulierten Kriterien wurde die Qualität der Evidenz für das Fehlen einer Beziehung zwischen PC-Arbeit und KTS als moderat eingestuft

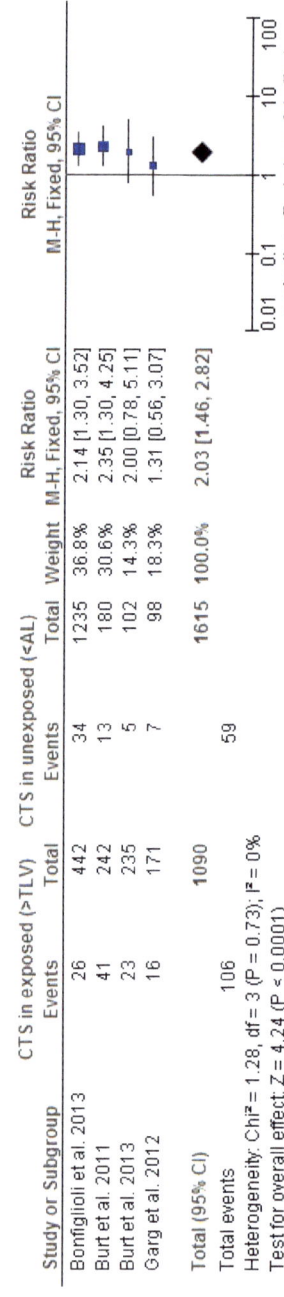

Study or Subgroup	CTS in exposed (>AL<TLV)		CTS in unexposed (<AL)			Risk Ratio	Risk Ratio
	Events	Total	Events	Total	Weight	M-H, Fixed, 95% CI	M-H, Fixed, 95% CI
Bonfiglioli et al. 2013	24	518	34	1235	61.6%	1.68 [1.01, 2.81]	
Burt et al. 2011	3	23	13	180	9.0%	1.81 [0.56, 5.87]	
Burt et al. 2013	1	10	5	102	2.7%	2.04 [0.26, 15.79]	
Garg et al. 2012	12	160	7	98	26.6%	1.05 [0.43, 2.58]	
Total (95% CI)		**711**		**1615**	**100.0%**	**1.54 [1.02, 2.31]**	
Total events	40		59				

Heterogeneity: Chi² = 0.96, df = 3 (P = 0.81); I² = 0%
Test for overall effect: Z = 2.06 (P = 0.04)

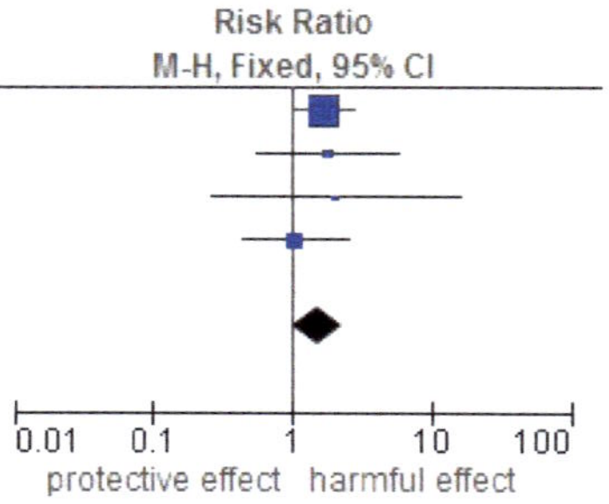

Abbildung 13 Forest plot – TLV für HAL: unter dem Aktionslimit (AL) vs. über dem Aktionslimit und bis zum Grenzschwellenwert (TLV)

Study or Subgroup	CTS in exposed (>TLV)		CTS in unexposed (<AL)			Risk Ratio	Risk Ratio
	Events	Total	Events	Total	Weight	M-H, Fixed, 95% CI	M-H, Fixed, 95% CI
Bonfiglioli et al. 2013	26	442	34	1235	36.8%	2.14 [1.30, 3.52]	
Burt et al. 2011	41	242	13	180	30.6%	2.35 [1.30, 4.25]	
Burt et al. 2013	23	235	5	102	14.3%	2.00 [0.78, 5.11]	
Garg et al. 2012	16	171	7	98	18.3%	1.31 [0.56, 3.07]	
Total (95% CI)		**1090**		**1615**	**100.0%**	**2.03 [1.46, 2.82]**	
Total events	106		59				

Heterogeneity: Chi² = 1.28, df = 3 (P = 0.73); I² = 0%
Test for overall effect: Z = 4.24 (P < 0.0001)

Abbildung 14 Forest Plot – TLV für HAL: unter dem Aktionslimit (AL) vs. über dem Grenzschwellenwert (TLV)

2.4.4 Evaluationsstudie – belastende Körperhaltungen in der Altenpflege reduzieren

Sechs Monate nach der Intervention konnte der Zeitanteil (Median) in sagittalen Neigungen über 20° um 29% statistisch signifikant reduziert werden (von 1772 auf 1708 Rumpfbeugungen pro Schicht). Der Zeitanteil stark ausgeprägter Rumpfneigungen (>60°) konnte um 60% signifikant verringert werden (von 288 auf 135). Statische Körperhaltungen (>20°/≥4 Sek.) wurden signifikant um 22% reduziert (von 462 auf 329). Die Zeit in sagittalen Neigungen über 20° wurde um 27 Minuten pro Schicht verringert (detaillierte Ergebnisse siehe Tabelle 4, Publikation 4).

Die Ergebnisse der Videoanalyse zeigten, dass insgesamt 217 Basis-Pflegetätigkeiten am Bett beobachtet wurden. Davon wurde, wie im Seminar empfohlen, in 44,7% der Pflegesituationen das Bett hüfthoch angepasst. In 44,2% der Pflegesituationen wurde das Bett nur teilweise und in 11,1% gar nicht erhöht. Insgesamt wurden 52 Pflegesituationen im Bad beobachtet; in 67,3% wurden die Grundpflegetätigkeiten in einer sitzenden Position durchgeführt. Zusammen betrachtet wurden die ergonomischen Maßnahmen in 49% aller Pflegesituationen korrekt angewendet.

Die Telefoninterviews ergaben, dass alle Probanden ihre ungünstigen Haltungen während der Arbeit bewusster wahrnahmen. Die Mehrheit (96%) achtete häufiger darauf, das Bett auf die empfohlene Höhe anzupassen. 50% der Probanden gaben an, dass Zeitdruck und Arbeitsstress sie daran hinderten, das Bett entsprechend anzupassen. Mehr als 90% achteten vermehrt auf ergonomische Methoden zur Mobilisierung der Pflegebedürftigen im Bett. Die Mehrheit gestaltete das Bewohnerzimmer ergonomisch um, sodass z. B. häufig benötigte Utensilien in eine ergonomische Höhe umgelagert wurden. Des Weiteren verwendeten alle das Pflegekörbchen für die häufig gebrauchten Pflegeutensilien. Jeweils 64% verwendeten den Wäschekorb und einen Pflegehocker im Bad. Lediglich 14% berichteten von Umsetzungsschwierigkeiten. Die häufigsten Gründe waren Zeitdruck aufgrund von Personalmangel, andere Prioritäten auf der Station oder andere Wünsche des Bewohners.

2.5 Diskussion

Diese kumulative Arbeit beschreibt die Häufigkeit von MSB in bestimmten Berufsgruppen, stellt die wissenschaftliche Evidenz für den Zusammenhang zwischen beruflichen Belastungsfaktoren und MSE am Beispiel des KTS zusammen und zeigt in einer Interventionsstudie Möglichkeiten zur Vermeidung beruflicher Belastungsfaktoren für MSB am Beispiel der ungünstigen Körperhaltungen in der Altenpflege auf. Für Tierärzte und Auszubildende wurde gezeigt, dass die Prävalenz von MSE/MSB hoch ist. Ferner konnten mögliche Zusammenhänge zwischen beruflichen Belastungen und MSB der oberen Extremitäten bei Tierärzten aufgezeigt werden. In einer vertieften Analyse der Literatur erwiesen sich unabhängig von der Berufsgruppe Repetition, Kraftaufwand und Vibration als arbeitsbedingte Risikofaktoren für das KTS. In einer Interventionsstudie wurde festgestellt, dass statische Körperhaltungen sowie häufige Oberkörperneigungen, die als Risikofaktoren für Rückenbeschwerden angenommen werden, durch relativ einfache ergonomische Maßnahmen in der Altenpflege reduziert werden können. Diese Maßnahmen könnten daher zur Reduktion vom MSB bei Pflegekräften beitragen, was in weiteren Studien zu überprüfen wäre.

Epidemiologische Erkenntnisse lassen zum einen Rückschlüsse auf beruflich und gesundheitlich belastete Kollektive zu und zum anderen ermöglichen sie eine Identifizierung und Quantifizierung von Expositionsfaktoren sowie die Abschätzung des Erkrankungsrisikos bei definierten Expositionen. Der epidemiologische Erkenntnisgewinn im Hinblick auf die arbeitsbezogenen Risikofaktoren und ihren Einfluss auf die Entstehung von MSE/MSB in den jeweiligen Berufen ist mit Vorsicht zu deuten, da vielfältige Faktoren eine Rolle spielen. Im Folgenden werden die Ergebnisse der hier vorgelegten vier Studien im Kontext der wissenschaftlichen Literatur kritisch diskutiert und ihre methodischen Stärken und Schwächen hervorgehoben. Eine ausführliche Diskussion der Ergebnisse kann den einzelnen Publikationen entnommen werden.

2.5.1 Empirische Studie – Muskel-Skelett-Beschwerden bei Veterinären in Deutschland

Die mittels Selbsteinschätzung durchgeführte Studie zu MSB und funktionellen körperlichen Einschränkungen wurde zum ersten Mal unter Veterinären in Deutschland durchgeführt. Im internationalen Vergleich ist sie die größte ihrer

Art in dieser Berufsgruppe. In Übereinstimmung mit der internationalen Literatur wird zum einen deutlich, dass MSB der oberen Extremitäten in dieser Berufsgruppe häufig vorkommen (Scuffham et al. 2010b; Smith et al. 2009) und zum anderen, dass Großtierpraktiker häufiger über MSB der distalen oberen Extremitäten klagten (Gabel & Gerberich 2002; Norwood et al. 2000). Arbeitsbedingte Unfälle wurden überwiegend von Großtierpraktikern angegeben. An Unfällen, die zu Verletzungen oder Beschwerden an den distalen Extremitäten führten, waren vorwiegend Tiere beteiligt. Eine nicht unerhebliche Anzahl der Befragten hatte so starke Beschwerden, dass sie an mindestens sieben Tagen in den vorausgegangenen 12 Monaten funktionelle Einschränkungen erlebten. Dieser Aspekt ist von Bedeutung, da dadurch die Ausübung der beruflichen Tätigkeit nur eingeschränkt möglich ist. Dieser Ausfall kann bei überwiegend selbstständigen Veterinären Gewinneinbußen oder im schlimmsten Fall einen vorzeitigen Berufsausstieg zur Folge haben. Abgesehen davon können Schmerzen und funktionelle körperliche Beeinträchtigung die Lebensqualität der Betroffenen erheblich mindern. Studien mit zusätzlichen bildgebenden oder diagnostischen Verfahren diagnostizieren allerdings deutlich seltener Erkrankungen des Bewegungsapparates (Lee et al. 2001; Toomingas et al. 1995). Da sich die für die Prävention zugänglichen Frühformen selten auf reliable Parameter stützen, schlagen Hartmann und Spallek (2009) vor, neben der körperlichen Untersuchung auch Funktionsstörungen für die auszuführende Arbeit zu bestimmen. Also wurde angestrebt, die durch MSB hervorgerufenen funktionellen Beeinträchtigungen im Alltag als abhängige Variable einzubeziehen.

Höheres Alter, Geschlecht, frühere Verletzungen, BMI, Praxistyp, Veterinärverfahren wie zahnmedizinische Eingriffe, Rektaluntersuchungen, Geburtshilfe sowie hohe quantitative Anforderungen und Burnout erhöhten die Wahrscheinlichkeit von funktionellen Einschränkungen. Die gefundene Beziehung zwischen Alter und MSB bestätigt die Ergebnisse anderer Untersuchungen (Randall et al. 2012; Scuffham et al. 2010b). Aus physiologischer Sicht ist dies zu erwarten, da mit steigendem Alter die Belastbarkeit des Stütz- und Bewegungsapparates abnimmt (de Zwart et al. 1995). Die beobachteten geschlechtsspezifischen Unterschiede lassen vermuten, dass unterschiedliche Tätigkeitsfelder hierbei eine Rolle spielen. Berry et al. (2012) berichten, dass CTD auslösende Tätigkeiten von beiden Geschlechtern unterschiedlich eingeschätzt wurden. Männer sahen die häufigen Rektalpalpationen und Geburtshilfe als risikobehaftete Tätigkeiten für ihre CTD, Frauen hingegen den häufigen Gebrauch von Utensilien oder Computerarbeit.

Die veterinären Diagnostik- und Behandlungsprozeduren können eine entscheidende Rolle bei der Entstehung oder Verschlimmerung von Symptomen spielen. Scuffham et al. (2010a) befragten Veterinäre zu Routineuntersuchungen, die möglicherweise MSB begünstigten. Groß- und Gemischttierpraktiker gaben an, dass insbesondere Rektaluntersuchungen, Geburtshilfe, Ultraschalluntersuchungen sowie Huf- und Lahmheitsdiagnostik risikobehaftete Tätigkeiten für MSB seien. Kleintierpraktiker hingegen empfanden das Heben und Tragen sowie chirurgische Eingriffe als belastend. In einer anderen Studie wurde berichtet, dass bei Großtierpraktikern akute traumatische Verletzungen und CTD überwiegend mit Rektaluntersuchungen zusammenhingen (Cattell 2000). Fallberichte verweisen darauf, dass multiple Rektaluntersuchungen möglicherweise mit neurologischen Störungen in den Versorgungsgebieten der Nervi medianus, ulnares und radiales sowie mit Impingement-Symptomen an der HWS (C5–C7) im Zusammenhang stehen (Ailsby 1996; Singleton 2005). Der gefundene Zusammenhang zwischen MSB der oberen Extremitäten und dem Tätigkeitsprofil scheint also plausibel zu sein. Mit der vorliegenden Prävalenzstudie konnte zwar das Ausmaß des Gesundheitsproblems quantifiziert und mögliche Zusammenhänge zwischen beruflicher Exposition und dem Auftreten von MSB abgeschätzt werden, jedoch lassen sich keine kausalen Schlussfolgerungen ableiten. Hierzu sind Studien mit prospektivem Design, längeren Beobachtungszeiträumen und der Erfassung von relevanten Confoundern erforderlich. Die daraus gewonnenen Erkenntnisse würden bei der Ermittlung und Beurteilung der Exposition im BK-Verfahren eine evidenzbasierte Entscheidungshilfe liefern. Eine weiterführende Betrachtung dieser beobachteten Zusammenhänge und die Entwicklung und Umsetzung von Präventionsmaßnahmen ist angebracht, denn diese Berufsgruppe ist bei der BGW in die höchste Gefahrenklasse[13] eingruppiert (BGW 2012). Außerdem ist davon auszugehen, dass durch den demografischen Wandel und den Nachwuchsmangel in der Veterinärmedizin, die Berufsverweildauer weiter steigen und somit der Anteil älterer Beschäftigter zunehmen wird (Kostelnik & Heuwieser 2009). Auch dieser Umstand unterstreicht die Wichtigkeit präventiver Maßnahmen, insbesondere für ältere Beschäftigte. Das Querschnittsdesign eignet sich nur begrenzt, um praxistaugliche Empfehlungen zu generieren. Folglich werden an dieser Stelle keine konkreten Maßnahmen formuliert. Dennoch sollten tierärztliche Verbände

---

[13] Die Gefahrenklassen werden anhand der Anzahl der Arbeits- und Wegeunfälle, BK-Meldungen und Höhe der Rehabilitationsleistungen ermittelt.

und Versicherungsorgane ihren Mitgliedern Schulungen und Informationen zum sicheren Umgang mit Tieren und der Ausrüstung zur Verfügung stellen. Solche Schulungen könnten bereits in das Curriculum für angehende Veterinäre einfließen.

2.5.2 Empirische Studie – Gesundheitszustand, -verhalten und Perspektiven von Auszubildenden in pflegerischen und sozialen Berufen

In der vorliegenden Studie wurden erstmalig in vergleichender Weise der Gesundheitszustand, das Gesundheitsverhalten sowie berufliche Zukunftsperspektiven von Auszubildenden in pflegerischen und sozialen Berufen beschrieben. Verglichen mit den Auszubildenden aus anderen Berufsgruppen trieben Altenpflegeschüler seltener Sport, rauchten häufiger und wiesen ein ungünstiges Ernährungsverhalten auf. Auszubildende in der GuK zeigten gegenüber anderen Berufen insgesamt ein besseres Gesundheitsverhalten. Alkohol wurde in allen Gruppen einheitlich stark konsumiert. Der Anteil übergewichtiger oder adipöser Auszubildender lag bei über 30%. Mehr als ein Drittel litt bereits an psychischen Erkrankungen oder MSE. Mit zunehmenden Lehrjahren zeigten Auszubildende eine stärker ausgeprägte Irritation, geringere Arbeitszufriedenheit sowie einen verminderten Wunsch, im jeweiligen Beruf zu bleiben. Die höchsten Werte hatten Auszubildende in der Erziehung/SPA. Analog dazu wollte die Mehrheit diesen Beruf auch in den kommenden Jahren ausüben. Bei den Altenpflegeschülern waren es die Hälfte und in der GuK lediglich 36%.

Die vergleichende Gesamtschau des Gesundheitszustandes und -verhaltens sowie Zukunftsperspektiven von Auszubildenden geht teilweise über die Zielsetzung dieser Synopse hinaus. Demzufolge wird in der nachfolgenden Diskussion der Fokus auf die gewonnenen Erkenntnisse zu MSE gelegt. Ein nicht unerheblicher Anteil gab an, in den vorangegangenen zwölf Monaten unter MSE gelitten zu haben. Hohe Prävalenzen von MSE stellten auch andere Studien bei Pflegeschülern und Beschäftigten in der Erziehung fest. In diesen berichteten zwischen 25% und 53% von MSE oder MSB (McGrath & Huntington 2007; Mitchell et al. 2010; Schwanke et al. 2011). Auszubildende im Alter zwischen 23 und 26 Jahren hatten eine etwa dreifach höhere Wahrscheinlichkeit, an MSE zu leiden als Auszubildende in der jüngsten Alterskategorie (<19 Jahre). Bei Auszubildenden im Alter von 27 bis 30 Jahren lag jedoch keine erhöhte Wahrscheinlichkeit für MSE vor, sodass hier kein konsistenter Alterseffekt beobachtet wurde. Andere Untersuchungen bestätigen einen Alterstrend (Bot et al. 2005; de Zwart et al. 1997). Es ist nicht auszuschließen, dass dieses Ergebnis durch die eng gefasste Einstufung der Alterskategorien zustande kam. Außerdem zeigten Auszubildende bei Vorliegen einer psychischen Beeinträchtigung eine erhöhte Wahrscheinlichkeit für MSE. Die Kausalitätsrichtung ist hier allerdings unklar. Lewinsohn et al. (1998) stellten fest, dass körperliche Erkrankungen signifikante Risikofaktoren für eine Depression bei älteren Jugendlichen sind. Hogg-Johnson et al. (2008) wiederum gehen von einer hohen Evidenz für eine Wechselwirkung zwischen körperlichen und psychischen Erkrankungen aus. Ein niedriger sozioökonomischer Status (SES) erwies sich im univariaten Modell als Schutzfaktor für MSE. In der Literatur finden sich für diesen Zusammenhang inkonsistente Ergebnisse. In einem Review schlussfolgern die Autoren, dass mehrere Studien auf eine inverse Beziehung zwischen SES und MSE hindeuteten (McBeth & Jones 2007). Gründe für die inkonsistenten Ergebnisse können möglicherweise die verschiedenen Methoden zur Erfassung des SES sein oder dieser korreliert mit anderen Risikofaktoren, die mit MSE im Zusammenhang stehen. Des Weiteren wurde im univariaten, jedoch nicht im multivariaten Modell gezeigt, dass Arbeitszufriedenheit mit MSE zusammenhängt. Demgegenüber wurde in einer Übersichtsarbeit für die Beziehung zwischen Kreuzschmerzen und Arbeitszufriedenheit eine hohe Evidenz gefunden (Hoogendoorn et al. 2000). In dieser Arbeit konnten keine der gesundheitsrelevanten Verhaltensweisen mit MSE in Beziehung gebracht werden. Zum einen kann dies an der kleinen Stichprobe in den einzelnen Gruppen liegen und zum anderen können weitere Faktoren, die hier nicht berücksichtigt wurden, die Entwicklung von MSE mitbeeinflussen. Aufgrund einer Querschnittsbetrachtung von Zusammenhängen ist die Interpretation der Ergebnisse nur eingeschränkt möglich. Mögliche Verzerrungen durch falsche Angaben oder sozial erwünschte Antworten sollten als weitere wesentliche Limitation betont werden. Des Weiteren kann aufgrund der Gelegenheitsstichprobe keine statistische Repräsentativität gewährleistet werden.

Obgleich einige methodische Schwächen vorliegen, implizieren die vorliegenden Ergebnisse, dass gut strukturierte Lehrinhalte, die auf die Stärkung der eigenen Gesundheit und die Vermeidung von Risikofaktoren abzielen, für alle Ausbildungsberufe von Vorteil wären. Der hohe Tabakkonsum unter den Schülern verdeutlicht den Bedarf an individuellen Beratungsangeboten oder einer berufsschulübergreifenden Antiraucherpolitik. Nicht zuletzt wird angenommen, dass die Integration stressreduzierender Maßnahmen auf Verhaltens- und/oder Verhältnisebene den Konsum von Tabak und auch Alkohol wirksam vermindern könnten.

Zur frühzeitigen Vorbeugung von Beschwerden des Muskel-Skelett-Systems bedarf es an Unterstützungsangeboten für rücken- und gelenkschonende Arbeitsweisen sowie flächendeckende Bereitstellung von kleinen Hilfsmitteln. Ein aktiver und gesunder Lebensstil ist ebenso nicht zu vernachlässigen, denn dadurch kann das Muskel-Skelett-System nachhaltig gestärkt und somit mögliche Verletzungen und Erkrankung im Arbeitsalltag verhindert oder zumindest reduziert werden.

2.5.3 Systematisches Overview über Systematische Reviews und eine Meta-Analyse – berufsbedingtes KTS

Dieses Overview und Update der aktuellen Primärliteratur bestätigt aus epidemiologischer Sicht den Zusammenhang zwischen beruflichen biomechanischen Risikofaktoren und der Entstehung von KTS. Die Klärung dieser Beziehung hilft bei der Beurteilung von KTS im BK-Verfahren sowie bei der Entwicklung von Strategien zur Reduzierung oder Vermeidung von beruflichen Belastungen. Für Repetition, Kraftaufwand sowie kombinierte Belastungen kann von einer hohen Qualität der Evidenz ausgegangen werden. Die Qualität der Evidenz für den Zusammenhang zwischen Vibration und KTS kann als moderat und für nicht neutrale Handpositionen als gering beurteilt werden. Eine Verursachung von KTS durch Computerarbeit ist aus epidemiologischer Perspektive unzureichend gesichert. Ein weiteres Ergebnis ist der Nachweis einer Dosis-Wirkung-Beziehung zwischen der kumulativen beruflichen Exposition gegenüber Repetition und Kraftaufwand. Bereits ab einem mäßigen HAL-TLV-Wert ist das Risiko für KTS geringfügig, aber signifikant erhöht. Bei Überschreiten des HAL-TLV-Wertes verdoppelt sich das Risiko.

Es besteht eine hohe Konsistenz für die Faktoren Repetition, Kraftaufwand und Vibration, die auch unter Berücksichtigung unterschiedlicher Berufsgruppen, Messmethoden und KTS-Falldefinitionen bestätigt wird. Zwischen nicht neutralen Handpositionen und KTS zeigt sich eine schwache Konsistenz. Die epidemiologische Evidenz von Flexion/Extension als unabhängige Risikofaktoren für KTS wurde in einem NIOSH-Review als unzureichend eingestuft. In Kombination mit anderen Belastungsfaktoren wird jedoch ein möglicher kausaler Zusammenhang vermutet (Bernard 1997). Um sichere Expositionslevel für Flexion/Extension ableiten zu können, werden valide konsistente Ergebnisse zur Intensität, Dauer und Häufigkeit aus epidemiologischen Studien benötigt. Eine plausible Erklärung liefern experimentelle und klinische Studien. Diesen zufolge wird durch extreme chronische

Flexionshaltung und Hyperextension der Druck im Karpaltunnel erheblich erhöht, wodurch der N. medianus gegen das Karpaltunneldach gepresst wird. Als Folge kann, zumindest kurzzeitig, eine Funktionsbeeinträchtigung des Nervs auftreten (Viikari-Juntura & Silverstein 1999). Im Hinblick auf die PC-Arbeit wurden inkonsistente Ergebnissen gefunden. Ein Overview schlussfolgerte, dass zwar eine hohe Evidenz für akute Schmerzen bei intensiver Nutzung bestehe, die Evidenz für die Entwicklung von spezifischen Krankheitsbildern oder chronischen Schmerzen jedoch unzureichend sei (Andersen et al. 2011).

Ab einer Verdopplung des Risikos kann von einer vorwiegend beruflichen Verursachung einer Erkrankung ausgegangen werden (SGB VII, § 9, Ziffer 8.2); dies entspricht einem ätiologischen Anteil von über 50% bei exponierten Personen. Mit Ausnahme der Exposition gegenüber PC-Arbeit besteht bei allen Faktoren mindestens eine Verdopplung des Risikos.

Ein Kausalzusammenhang ist dann plausibel, wenn der Erkrankungsbeginn in einem unmittelbaren zeitlichen Zusammenhang mit der Exposition steht. Die meisten SRs hatten jedoch überwiegend Studien mit Fall-Kontroll- und Querschnittsdesign eingeschlossen. Lozano-Calderon et al. (2008) zeigten, dass mehr als 80% der untersuchten Studien den Zeitaspekt nicht beschrieben haben. Lediglich drei bis vier prospektive Studien wurden in qualitativ gute SRs eingeschlossen. Darauf beruhend kann eine Kausalität hinsichtlich der beobachteten Assoziation nicht gänzlich hergestellt werden (Barcenilla et al. 2012; van Rijn et al. 2009). Durch den Einschluss von weiteren Primärstudien konnte jedoch ein positiver zeitlicher Zusammenhang beobachtet werden.

In Bezug auf die Expositionsdauer zeigte eine gepoolte Analyse mit einem Sieben-Jahre-Follow-up, dass Werktätige, die weniger als 3,5 Jahre im selben Job arbeiteten, eine höhere Inzidenzrate aufwiesen als solche, die bereits länger tätig waren (Harris-Adamson et al. 2013). Eine weitere prospektive Studie verdeutlichte, dass bereits eine kurze Exposition von sechs Monaten in Berufen mit hoher Repetition und hohem Kraftaufwand mit erhöhter KTS-Inzidenz assoziiert war (Evanoff et al. 2014). Folglich kann eine Expositionsdauer von bis zu drei Jahren bereits ausreichen, um ein beruflich erworbenes KTS zu entwickeln. Aus den Studien kann jedoch nicht der Schluss gezogen werden, dass eine längere Exposition gegen einen Ursachenzusammenhang spricht.

Ergebnisse zu Dosis-Wirkung-Beziehungen konnten aus den SRs nicht sicher abgeleitet werden und deshalb wurde die aktuelle Literatur daraufhin überprüft. Durch die Verwendung der ACGIH-Grenzwerte wurde ein signifikanter Trend für HAL und KTS nachgewiesen. Frühere Untersuchungen beobachteten ebenfalls einen monotonen Risikoanstieg zwischen kombinierten Expositionen und KTS-Prävalenz und -Inzidenz (Franzblau et al. 2005; Violante et al. 2007). Eine Analyse mit gepoolten Originaldaten zeigte zwar eine Risikoerhöhung für Expositionen über dem Aktionslimit (HR 1,7; 95%-KI 1,2–2,5), jedoch keinen weiteren Risikoanstieg über dem Schwellenwert (HR 1,5; 95%-KI 1,0–2,1) (Kapellusch et al. 2014). Im Einklang mit anderen Studien verdeutlichen diese Ergebnisse, dass derzeitige ACGIH-Grenzwerte für das Aktionslimit nicht hinreichend protektiv sind und daher überdacht werden sollten (Bonfiglioli et al. 2013; Kapellusch et al. 2014).

Eine Meta-Regressionsanalyse zeigte, dass unterschiedliche KTS-Falldefinitionen, Studiendesigns, methodische Schwächen sowie Untersuchungsländer signifikant zur Aufklärung der Heterogenität beitrugen (Barcenilla et al. 2012). Studien mit weniger stringenten Kriterien (z. B. nur Symptomerfassung) wiesen häufiger einen Zusammenhang, höhere Prävalenzen und Inzidenzen nach als solche mit einer konservativen Falldefinition (Lozano-Calderon et al. 2008). Mögliche Folge könnte eine Überdiagnostizierung oder Fehlklassifikation des KTS in epidemiologischen Studien sein. Die Kombination aus positivem NLG-Test und Symptomen lieferten die präzisesten Ergebnisse (Rempel et al. 1998). Ebenso problematisch war die mangelnde Verwendung von objektiven Messverfahren zur Expositionserfassung. Oft wurde die Häufigkeit und Dauer der Exposition retrospektiv über Selbstangaben bestimmt, was zu einer möglichen Fehlklassifikation und Verzerrung durch hohe Effektstärken führte.

Die Validität eines Overviews hängt letztlich von der Validität der eingeschlossenen SRs und Primärstudien sowie der angewandten Auswahl- und Bewertungsprozesse ab. Eine wesentliche Limitation besteht darin, dass die extrahierte Information aus den SRs bereits durch andere Autoren gefiltert und aufgearbeitet wurde. Da bisher formale Kriterien für die Bewertung der Qualität der Evidenz für Overviews fehlen, wurde ein qualitativer Ansatz gewählt, indem die Studienvalidität und Konsistenz der Ergebnisse als Kernkriterien definiert wurden. Bei dieser Form der Evidenzsynthese stellt die Überlappung der Studienpools ein Problem dar. In dieser Untersuchung war die Überschneidungsquote mit einem CCA-Wert von 13,3 hoch und bedeutet, dass hier eine Doppelzählung der Evidenz vorliegt. Dadurch kann die Validität erheblich eingeschränkt sein. Außerdem wird darauf verwiesen, dass die Aktualität der SRs ein mögliches Problem darstellen kann (Pieper et al. 2013). Durch den Einschluss aktueller Studien konnte die Validität des Overviews jedoch gesteigert werden.

Abschließend wird empfohlen, dass künftige ätiologische Studien objektive Verfahren zur Expositionserfassung mit einer konservativen KTS-Definition verbinden. Die vorliegende Analyse bestätigt, dass KTS nach einem Nachweis beruflicher Risiken als BK anerkennungsfähig ist. Bei Zusammenhangsbegutachtungen im BK-Verfahren sollten neben beruflichen Expositionen auch andere Faktoren wie BMI oder Komorbiditäten berücksichtigt werden, da sie mit beruflichen Expositionsfaktoren interagieren können.

2.5.4 Evaluationsstudie – belastende Körperhaltungen in der Altenpflege reduzieren

Die Ergebnisse der messtechnischen Evaluation zeigen, dass ungünstige Körperneigungen und -haltungen durch zielgerichtete ergonomische Maßnahmen signifikant reduziert werden können. Demnach wurde während einer Arbeitsschicht die Zeit, die in einer vorgeneigten Haltung verbracht wurde (>20°) von zwei auf eineinhalb Stunden verringert. Lediglich bei der Hälfte aller Pflegetätigkeiten am Bett und im Bad wurden die Maßnahmen adäquat angewendet. Dieser Umstand impliziert, dass es bei konsequenter Anpassung des Bettes und Nutzung eines Hockers noch mehr Reduktionspotenzial bei ungünstigen Neigungen und Haltungen gibt. Die Teilnehmer empfanden Umfang und Inhalt des Seminars als hilfreich und angemessen. Dabei ist allerdings zu berücksichtigen, dass dieses Seminar nicht primär darauf abzielte, Rückenbeschwerden zu reduzieren, sondern Pflegekräfte für die häufigen und oft verkannten Neigungen und Haltungen zu sensibilisieren. Diese werden als zusätzliche Risikofaktoren für die Entwicklung von Rückenbeschwerden bei Pflegekräften diskutiert. Laut mehreren SRs liegt für diese Beziehung jedoch eine widersprüchliche Evidenzlage vor (Bakker et al. 2009; Ribeiro et al. 2012). Weitere Reviews unter Verwendung von Bradford-Hill-Kriterien für Kausalität machen ebenfalls deutlich, dass Körperhaltungen keine unabhängigen Risikofaktoren für Rückenschmerzen darstellen (Roffey et al. 2010; Wai et al. 2010). Wenngleich die epidemiologische Evidenzlage strittig ist, zeigen biomechanische experimentelle Untersuchungen, dass diese Bewegungsmuster unverhältnismäßige Belastungen auf das Muskel-Skelett-System ausüben (Olson et al. 2004;

Solomonow 2004; Solomonow et al. 2004). Bei sagittalen Oberkörperneigungen lässt die Aktivität der autochthonen Rückenmuskulatur nach. Die Hauptfunktion dieser Muskelgruppe liegt in der Aufrichtung und Stabilisierung der Wirbelsäule. Bei ausgeprägter Flexion des Oberkörpers ist die neuronale Aktivität der Streckmuskulatur erheblich vermindert, dieser Zustand wird auch als „myoelektrische Stille" beschrieben. In dieser Position lastet das Gewicht des Oberkörpers auf den sogenannten „passiven Strukturen" des Bewegungsapparates, den Bändern und Bandscheiben. Die Folge ist eine Reduktion der lumbalen Stabilität und durch den Nachweis von Spasmen entstehen auch mikrostrukturelle Schäden am viskoelastischen Gewebe (Olson et al. 2004; 2009). Die Autoren schlussfolgern, dass statische sowie zyklische lumbale Flexion ohne Lasten zusätzliche Risikofaktoren bei der Entwicklung von LWS-Erkrankungen darstellen (Olson et al. 2004; Solomonow et al. 2004). Wai et al. (2010) vermuten, dass die inkonsistenten Ergebnisse aus epidemiologischen Studien zum einen durch unterschiedliche ergonomische Bewertungen der Körperhaltungen und zum anderen durch unterschiedliche Definitionen des Outcomes herrühren. Das wird bereits deutlich, wenn die vorliegenden Ergebnisse mit anderen Monitoring-Studien in der Altenpflege verglichen werden. Beim ersten Messzeitpunkt verbrachten Pflegekräfte in unserer Untersuchung im Durchschnitt 36% der Arbeitszeit in vorgeneigter Haltung. Andere Untersuchungen stellten zum Teil stark abweichende Zeitanteile fest. Jansen et al. (2001) und Hodder et al. (2010) verwendeten in ihren Untersuchungen Neigungssensoren. Sie zeigten, dass 21% der Zeit in einer Winkelstellung von über 20° beziehungsweise 25% bei über 30° verbracht wurden. Ribeiro et al. (2011) nutzten einen sogenannten Wirbelsäulen-Beschleunigungswinkelmesser (Spineangle accelerometer) und fanden heraus, dass lediglich 5% der Zeit in vorgeneigter Haltung über 30° verbracht wurden. Diese Unterschiede beruhen wahrscheinlich auf den verschiedenen Messinstrumenten und dem Befestigungsort am Körper (z. B. an der BWS und/oder LWS). Abgesehen davon berichten mehrere Studien über Pflegepersonal von einer positiven Beziehung zwischen ungünstigen Körperhaltungen und der Entwicklung von Rückenbeschwerden (Jansen et al. 2004; Josephson et al. 1998; Yip 2004). Die Evidenzlage für diesen Zusammenhang ist jedoch spärlich; weitere Untersuchungen sind nötig, um eine Beziehung zwischen ungünstigen Körperhaltungen und Schäden am Muskel-Skelett-System nachzuweisen.

Diverse Studien belegen, dass Pflegekräfte einen bedeutenden Zeitanteil mit patientenfernen Aktivitäten verbringen (z. B. Betten machen, Aufräumen) und grundlegende Pflegetätigkeiten verrichten (Engels et al. 1994; Fiedler et al. 2012; Freitag et al. 2007; Hodder et al. 2010; Holmes et al. 2010). Eine einseitige Fokussierung auf Hebe- und Tragevorgänge würde somit eine deutliche Unterschätzung der körperlichen Gesamtbelastung in der Pflege zur Folge haben.

Der Vorteil dieser Evaluation liegt darin, dass hier ein objektives messtechnisches Verfahren in Verbindung mit Videoaufnahmen verwendet wurde. Somit konnte jeder Bewegung auch die entsprechende Tätigkeit zugeordnet werden. Ebenfalls sollten einige Schwächen erwähnt werden, die die Aussagekraft dieser Studie limitieren. Erstens: Die Ergebnisse können nicht uneingeschränkt auf alle Altenpflegekräfte übertragen werden, da es sich um keine Zufallsstichprobe handelt und die Probandenzahl aufgrund des logistischen Aufwandes begrenzt war. Zweitens: Das Tragen des CUELA-Messsystems und die parallelen Videoaufnahmen trugen womöglich zu einer Verhaltensänderung der Probanden bei, um den erwarteten Ergebnissen zu entsprechen. Dieser Umstand wird in epidemiologischen Studien auch als Hawthrone effect bezeichnet. Demnach kann hier eine Unterschätzung der Häufigkeit und Dauer von sagittalen Neigungen vorliegen. Drittens: Die interne Validität ist aufgrund des Fehlens einer Kontrollgruppe gefährdet. Damit eine signifikante Verhaltensänderung auf das Seminar zurückgeführt werden kann, bedarf es einer zufällig ausgewählten Kontrollgruppe. Zum einen können dadurch die erwarteten Ursachen für Variabilität minimiert und somit die Präzision der Ergebnisse verbessert werden; zum anderen können alternative Erklärungsversuche ausgeschlossen sowie eine kausale Beziehung konstatiert werden.

Es wurde gezeigt, dass durch einen relativ geringen organisatorischen Aufwand und eine Informationsvermittlung ungünstige Körperhaltungen in der Altenpflege zumindest kurzfristig verringert werden können. Die konsequente Anpassung von höhenverstellbaren Betten oder die ergonomische Umgestaltung von Bewohnerzimmern kann maßgeblich dazu beitragen, die Vielzahl von belastenden Körperhaltungen auf ein notwendiges Maß zu reduzieren. Demnach impliziert diese Pilotstudie, dass die Wirksamkeit von ergonomischen Maßnahmen im pflegerischen Setting gesteigert werden kann, wenn Schulungsprogramme zusätzlich zu rückengerechten Transfer- und Umlagerungshilfen auch das Bewusstsein für die ungünstigen Körperneigungen und -haltungen bei Pflegekräften schärfen sowie eine verstärkte Nutzung von Hilfsmitteln propagieren.

3 Literaturverzeichnis

ACGIH (2002) *Threshold Limit Values for chemical substances and physical agents in the work environment. American Conference of Governmental Industrial Hygienists (ACGIH), ed., Cincinnati, OH.*

Ailsby RL. (1996) *Occupational arm, shoulder, and neck syndrome affecting large animal practitioners. Can Vet J; 37:411.*

Alexandre NM, de Moraes MA, Correa Filho HR, Jorge SA. (2001) *Evaluation of a program to reduce back pain in nursing personnel. Rev Saude Publica; 35: 356-61.*

Almstadt E, Gebauer G, Medjedovic I. (2012)
Arbeitsplatz Kita. Berufliche und gesundheitliche Belastungen von Beschäftigten in Kindertageseinrichtungen im Land Bremen, Institut Arbeit und Wirtschaft (IAW), ed., Schriftenreihe Nr. 15, http://www.iaw.uni-bremen.de/ccm/cms-service/stream/asset/IAW-Schriftenreihe15.pdf?asset_id=3296036 (Stand 31.01.2016).

Andersen JH, Fallentin N, Thomsen JF, Mikkelsen S. (2011)
Risk factors for neck and upper extremity disorders among computers users and the effect of interventions: an overview of systematic reviews. PLOS ONE; 6: e19691.

Anton D, Rosecrance J, Merlino L, Cook T. (2002) *Prevalence of musculoskeletal symptoms and carpal tunnel syndrome among dental hygienists. Am J Ind Med; 42: 248-57.*

Ariens GA, van Mechelen W, Bongers PM, Bouter LM, van der Wal G. (2001) *Psychosocial riskfactors for neck pain: a systematic review. Am J Ind Med; 39: 180-93.*

Aroori S, Spence RA. (2008) *Carpal tunnel syndrome. Ulster Med J; 77: 6-17.*

Assmus H, Antonidis G, Bischoff C, Haussmann P, Martini AK, Mascharka Z, Scheglmann K, Schwerdtfeger K, Selbmann HK, Towfigh H, Vogt T, Wessels KD, Wustner-Hofmann M. (2007) *Diagnosis and therapy of carpal tunnel syndrome--guideline of the German Societies of Handsurgery, Neurosurgery, Neurology, Orthopaedics, Clinical Neurophysiology and Functional Imaging, Plastic, Reconstructive and Aesthetic Surgery, and Surgery for Traumatology. Handchir Mikrochir Plast Chir; 39: 276-88.*

Bakker EW, Verhagen AP, van Trijffel E, Lucas C, Koes BW. (2009) *Spinal mechanical load as a risk factor for low back pain: a systematic review of prospective cohort studies. Spine (Phila Pa 1976); 34: E281-93.*

Balague F, Mannion AF, Pellise F, Cedraschi C. (2012) *Non-specific low back pain. Lancet; 379: 482-91.*

Baldwin D, Gaines S, Wold JL, Williams A, Leary J. (2007) *The health of female child care providers: implications for quality of care. J Community Health Nurs; 24: 1-17.*

Barcenilla A, March LM, Chen JS, Sambrook PN. (2012) *Carpal tunnel syndrome and its relationship to occupation: a meta-analysis. Rheumatology (Oxford); 51: 250-61.*

BAuA, Bundesanstalt für Arbeitsschutz und Arbeitsmedizin (2015) *Arbeitswelt im Wandel: Zahlen Daten – Fakten. http://www.baua.de/de/Publikationen/Broschueren/A92.html;jsessionid=23F40F87B68ECB9BB1409A23DC534388.1_cid343 (Stand 17.12.2015).*

Becker LA, Oxman AD. (2008) *Overviews of Reviews. In: Cochrane Handbook for Systematic Reviews of Interventions. ed. John Wiley & Sons, Ltd, 607-31.*

Behr T. (2015) *Aufbruch Pflege? Philosophischer Versuch einer Annäherung an das Faktische. In: Aufbruch Pflege – Hintergründe – Analysen – Entwicklungsperspektiven (Behr T, ed.). Springer: Wiesbaden, 17-22.*

Bernal D, Campos-Serna J, Tobias A, Vargas-Prada S, Benavides FG, Serra C. (2015) *Work-related psychosocial risk factors and musculoskeletal disorders in hospital nurses and nursing aides: A systematic review and meta-analysis. Int J Nurs Stud; 52: 635-48.*

Bernard BP. (1997) *Musculoskeletal disorders and workplace factors – a critical review of epidemiologicevidence for work-related musculoskeletal disorders of the neck, upper extremity, and low back, National Institute of Occupational Safety and Health (NIOSH), ed., http://www.cdc.gov/niosh/docs/97-141/pdfs/97-141.pdf (Stand 05.06.2014).*

Berry SL, Susitaival P, Ahmadi A, Schenker MB. (2012) *Cumulative trauma disorders among California veterinarians.Am J Ind Med; 55: 855-61.*

Best M. (1997) *An evaluation of Manutention training in preventing back strain and resultant injuriesinnurses. Safety Science; 25: 207-22.*

BGW, Berufsgenossenschaft für Gesundheitsdienst und Wohlfahrtspflege (2012) *Gefahrtarif der BGW. https://www.bgw-online.de/DE/Leistungen-Beitrag/Beitrag/Gefahrtarif/Gefahrtarif_node.html (Stand 27.01.2016).*

Bonfiglioli R, Mattioli S, Armstrong TJ, Graziosi F, Marinelli F, Farioli A, Violante FS. (2013) *Validation of the ACGIH TLV for hand activity level in the OCTOPUS cohort: a two-year longitudinal study of carpal tunnel syndrome. Scand J Work Environ Health; 39: 155-63.*

Bos EH, Krol B, Van Der Star A, Groothoff JW. (2006)*The effects of occupational interventions on reduction of musculoskeletal symptoms in the nursing profession. Ergonomics; 49:706-23.*

Bot SD, van der Waal JM, Terwee CB, van der Windt DA, Schellevis FG, Bouter LM, Dekker J. (2005) *Incidence and prevalence of complaints of the neck and upper extremity in general practice. Ann Rheum Dis; 64: 118-23.*

Burt S, Deddens JA, Crombie K, Jin Y, Wurzelbacher S, Ramsey J. (2013) *A prospective study of carpal tunnel syndrome: workplace and individual risk factors. Occup Environ Med; 70: 568-74.*

Camerino D, Conway PM, Van der Heijden BI, Estryn-Behar M, Consonni D, Gould D, Hasselhorn HM. (2006) *Low-perceived work ability, ageing and intention to leave nursing: a comparison among 10 European countries.J Adv Nurs; 56: 542-52.*

Caruso CC, Waters TR. (2008) *A review of work schedule issues and musculoskeletal disorders with an emphasis on the healthcare sector. Ind Health; 46: 523-34.*

Cattell M. (2000) *Rectal palpation associated cumulative trauma disorders and acute traumatic injury affecting bovine practitioners. Bovine practitioner; 34: 1-5.*

Coggon D, Ntani G, Vargas-Prada S, Martinez JM, Serra C, Benavides FG, Palmer KT. (2013) *International variation in absence from work attributed to musculoskeletal illness: findings from the CUPID study. Occup Environ Med; 70: 575-84.*

Cooper H, Koenka AC. (2012) *The overview of reviews: unique challenges and opportunities when research syntheses are the principal elements of new integrative scholarship. Am Psychol; 67: 446-62.*

Crary P. (2013) *Beliefs, behaviors, and health of undergraduate nursing students. Holist Nurs Pract; 27: 74-88.*

da Costa BR, Vieira ER. (2010) *Risk factors for work-related musculoskeletal disorders: A systematic review of recent longitudinal studies. Am J Ind Med; 53: 285-323.*

DAK, Deutsche Angestellten Krankenkasse (2015) *DAK – Gesundheitsreport 2015. http://www.dak.de/dak/gesundheit/DAK-Gesundheitsreport_2015-1587898.html (Stand 17.12.2015).*

Dathe D, Paul F, Stuth S. (2012) *Soziale Dienstleistungen: Steigende Arbeitslast trotz Personalzuwachs. WZBrief Arbeit; 12.*

Davis KG, Kotowski SE. (2015) *Prevalence of musculoskeletal disorders for nurses in hospitals, long-term care facilities, and home health care: a comprehensive review. Hum Factors; 57: 754-92.*

Dawson AP, McLennan SN, Schiller SD, Jull GA, Hodges PW, Stewart S. (2007) *Interventions to prevent back pain and back injury in nurses: a systematic review. Occup Environ Med; 64: 642-50.*

de Zwart BC, Frings-Dresen MH, van Dijk FJ. (1995) *Physical workload and the aging worker: a review of the literature. Int Arch Occup Environ Health; 68: 1-12.*

de Zwart BC, Broersen JP, Frings-Dresen MH, van Dijk FJ. (1997) *Musculoskeletal complaints in the Netherlands in relation to age, gender and physically demanding work. Int Arch Occup Environ Health; 70: 352-60.*

Deeks JJ, Higgins JPT, Altman DG. (2008) *Analysing Data and Undertaking Meta-Analyses. In: Cochrane Handbook for Systematic Reviews of Interventions. John Wiley & Sons, Ltd, 243-96.*

Dehlin O, Berg S, Andersson GB, Grimby G. (1981) *Effect of physical training and ergonomic counselling on the psychological perception of work and on the subjective assessment of low-back insufficiency. Scand J Rehabil Med; 13: 1-9.*

DESTATIS (2015) *Gesundheit – Personal 2013. Fachserie 12, Reihe 7.3.1., Statistisches Bundesamt, ed., Wiesbaden.*

DIN (2002) *Sicherheit von Maschinen – Menschliche körperliche Leistung – Teil 1: Begriffe. Deutsche Fassung EN 1005-1:2002-02. Deutsches Institut für Normung (DIN) e.V., ed., Beuth Verlag: Berlin.*

DIN (2005) *Sicherheit von Maschinen – Menschliche körperliche Leistung – Teil 4: Bewertung von Körperhaltungen und Bewegungen bei der Arbeit an Maschinen. Deutsche Fassung EN 1005-4:2005, Deutsches Institut für Normung e.V., ed., Beuth Verlag: Berlin.*

DRV, Deutsche Rentenversicherung Bund (2015) *Rentenversicherung in Zahlen 2015.* http://www.deutsche-rentenversicherung.de/cae/servlet/contentblob/238692/publication File/61815/01_rv_in_zahlen_2013.pdf *(Stand 15. 12. 2015).*

Ellegast R, Hermanns I, Schiefer C. (2009) *Workload assessment in field using the ambulatory CUELA system. In: Digital Human Modeling, Proceedings. 5620, (Duffy VG, ed.), Springer-Verlag: Berlin, 221-26.*

Engels JA, Landeweerd JA, Kant Y. (1994) *An OWAS-based analysis of nurses' working postures. Ergonomics; 37: 909-19.*

Engels JA, van der Gulden JW, Senden TF, Kolk JJ, Binkhorst RA. (1998) *The effects of an ergonomic-educational course. Postural load, perceived physical exertion, and biomechanical errors in nursing. Int Arch Occup Environ Health; 71: 336-42.*

Engkvist IL, Hjelm EW, Hagberg M, Menckel E, Ekenvall L. (2000) *Risk indicators for reported over-exertion back injuries among female nursing personnel. Epidemiology; 11: 519-22.*

Eriksen W, Bruusgaard D, Knardahl S. (2004) *Work factors as predictors of intense or disabling low back pain; a prospective study of nurses' aides. Occup Environ Med; 61: 398-404.*

Evanoff B, Zeringue A, Franzblau A, Dale AM. (2014) *Using job-title-based physical exposures from O*NET in an epidemiological study of carpal tunnel syndrome. Hum Factors; 56: 166-77.*

Fanello S, Frampas-Chotard V, Roquelaure Y, Jousset N, Delbos V, Jarny J, Penneau-Fontbonne D. (1999) *Evaluation of an educational low back pain prevention program for hospital employees. Rev Rhum Engl Ed; 66: 711-6.*

Fiedler KM, Weir PL, van Wyk PM, Andrews DM. (2012) *Analyzing what nurses do during work in a hospital setting: a feasibility study using video. Work; 43: 515-23.*

Franzblau A, Armstrong TJ, Werner RA, Ulin SS. (2005) *A cross-sectional assessment of the ACGIH TLV for hand activity level. Journal of occupational rehabilitation; 15: 57-67.*

Freitag S, Ellegast R, Dulon M, Nienhaus A. (2007) *Quantitative measurement of stressful trunk postures in nursing professions. Ann Occup Hyg; 51: 385-95.*

Freitag S, Fincke-Junod I, Seddouki R, Dulon M, Hermanns I, Kersten JF, Larsson TJ, Nienhaus A. (2012) *Frequent bending – an underestimated burden in nursing professions. Ann Occup Hyg; 56: 697-707.*

Freitag S, Seddouki R, Dulon M, Kersten JF, Larsson TJ, Nienhaus A. (2014) *The effect of working position on trunk posture and exertion for routine nursing tasks: an experimental study. Ann Occup Hyg; 58: 317-25.*

Fritschi L, Day L, Shirangi A, Robertson I, Lucas M, Vizard A. (2006) *Injury in Australian veterinarians. Occup Med (Lond); 56: 199-203.*

Gabel CL, Gerberich SG. (2002) *Risk factors for injury among veterinarians. Epidemiology; 13: 80-6.*

Garg A, Owen B. (1992) *Reducing back stress to nursing personnel: an ergonomic intervention in a nursing home. Ergonomics; 35: 1353-75.*

Giersiepen K, Spallek M. (2011) *Carpal tunnel syndrome as an occupational disease. Dtsch Arztebl Int; 108: 238-42.*

Glaser J, Höge T. (2005) *Probleme und Lösungen in der Pflege aus Sicht der Arbeits- und Gesundheitswissenschaften, Bundesanstalt für Arbeitsschutz und Arbeitsmedizin (BAuA), ed., http://www.baua.de/cae/servlet/contentblob/680434/publicationFile/47124/Gd18.pdf (Stand 31.01.2016).*

Gundewall B, Liljeqvist M, Hansson T. (1993) *Primary prevention of back symptoms and absence from work. A prospective randomized study amonghospital employees. Spine (Phila Pa 1976); 18: 587-94.*

Hagberg M, Morgenstern H, Kelsh M. (1992) *Impact of occupations and job tasks on the prevalence of carpal tunnel syndrome. Scand J Work Environ Health; 18: 337-45.*

Harling M, Strehmel P, Schablon A, Nienhaus A. (2009) *Psychosocial stress, demoralization and the consumption of tobacco, alcohol and medical drugs by veterinarians. J Occup Med Toxicol; 4: 4.*

Harris-Adamson C, Eisen EA, Dale AM, Evanoff B, Hegmann KT, Thiese MS, Kapellusch JM, Garg A, Burt S, Bao S, Silverstein B, Gerr F, Merlino L, Rempel D. (2013) *Personal and workplace psychosocial risk factors for carpal tunnel syndrome: a pooled study cohort. Occup Environ Med; 70: 529-37.*

Hartmann B, Spallek M. (2009) *Arbeitsbezogene Muskel-Skelett-Erkrankungen – Eine Gegenstandsbestimmung. Arbeitsmed Sozialmed Umweltmed; 8: 423-36.*

Hausmann C. (2009) *Burnout-Symptome bei österreichischen PflegeschülerInnen im dritten Ausbildungsjahr. Pflege; 22: 297-307.*

Hignett S. (2003) *Intervention strategies to reduce musculoskeletal injuries associated with handling patients: a systematic review. Occup Environ Med; 60: e6.*

Hirsch K, Voigt K, Gerlach K, Kugler J, Bergmann A. (2010) *Tabak-, Alkohol- und Drogenkonsum sowie Impfverhalten von Gesundheits- und KrankenpflegeschülerInnen in Sachsen-Anhalt. Heilberufe Science; 1: 127-32.*

Hodder JN, Holmes MW, Keir PJ. (2010) *Continuous assessment of work activities and posture in long-term care nurses. Ergonomics; 53: 1097-107.*

Hoehne-Hückstädt U, Herda C, Ellegast R, Hermanns I, Hamburger R, Ditchen D. (2007) *Muskel-Skelett-Erkrankungen der oberen Extremität und berufliche Tätigkeit. BGIA-Report 2/2007, Hauptverband der gewerblichen Berufsgenossenschaften (HVBG), ed., Sankt Augustin.*

Hoehne-Hückstädt U, Schedlbauer G, Hartmann B, Sander M, Spallek M, Zagrodnik F. (2014) *Carpal tunnel syndrome as an occupational disease. Zbl Arbeitsmed; 64: 113-16.*

Hoffmann SW, Tug S, Simon P. (2013) *Obesity prevalence and unfavorable health risk behaviors among German kindergarten teachers: cross-sectional results of the kindergarten teacher health study. BMC Public Health; 13: 927-27.*

Hogg-Johnson S, van der Velde G, Carroll LJ, Holm LW, Cassidy JD, Guzman J, Côté P, Haldeman S, Ammendolia C, Carragee E, Hurwitz E, Nordin M, Peloso P. (2008) *The burden and determinants of neck pain in the general population. Results of the Bone and Joint Decade 2000-2010 Task Force on Neck Pain and Its Associated Disorders. Spine; 3: 39-51.*

Holmes MWR, Hodder JN, Keir PJ. (2010) *Continuous assessment of low back loads in long-term care nurses. Ergonomics; 53: 1108-16.*

Holtermann A, Clausen T, Aust B, Mortensen OS, Andersen LL. (2013) *Risk for low back pain from different frequencies, load mass and trunk postures of lifting and carrying among female healthcare workers. Int Arch Occup Environ Health; 86: 463-70.*

Hoogendoorn WE, van Poppel MN, Bongers PM, Koes BW, Bouter LM. (2000) *Systematic review of psychosocial factors at work and private life as risk factors for back pain. Spine (Phila Pa 1976); 25: 2114-25.*

Horneij E, Hemborg B, Jensen I, Ekdahl C. (2001) *No significant differences between intervention programmes on neck, shoulder and low back pain: a prospective randomized study among home-care personnel. J Rehabil Med; 33: 170-6.*

Hoy D, Bain C, Williams G, March L, Brooks P, Blyth F, Woolf A, Vos T, Buchbinder R. (2012) *A systematic review of the global prevalence of low back pain. Arthritis Rheum; 64: 2028-37.*

ISO (2000) *Ergonomics – Evaluation of static working postures ISO 11226. Herausgegeben von ISO 11226:2000(E), i-18.15-12-2000. International Organization for Standardization ed., Geneva, Switzerland.*

Jansen JP, Burdorf A, Steyerberg E. (2001) *A novel approach for evaluating level, frequency and duration of lumbar posture simultaneously during work. Scand J Work Environ Health; 27: 373-80.*

Jansen JP, Morgenstern H, Burdorf A. (2004) *Dose-response relations between occupational exposures to physical and psychosocial factors and the risk of low back pain. Occup Environ Med; 61: 972-9.*

Josephson M, Vingård E, Group M-NS. (1998) *Workplace factors and care seeking for low-back pain among female nursing personnel. Scand J Work Environ Health; 24: 465-72.*

Kaminski A, Nauerth A, Pfefferle Pl. (2008) *Gesundheitszustand und Gesundheitsverhalten von Auszubildenden im ersten Lehrjahr – Erste Ergebnisse einer Befragung in Bielefelder Berufskollegs. Gesundheitswesen; 70: 38-46.*

Kapellusch JM, Gerr FE, Malloy EJ, Garg A, Harris-Adamson C, Bao SS, Burt SE, Dale AM, Eisen EA, Evanoff BA, Hegmann KT, Silverstein BA, Theise MS, Rempel DM. (2014) *Exposure-response relationships for the ACGIH threshold limit value for hand-activity level: results from a pooled data study of carpal tunnel syndrome. Scand J Work Environ Health; 40: 610-20.*

Kim SS, Okechukwu CA, Dennerlein JT, Boden Ll, Hopcia K, Hashimoto DM, Sorensen G. (2014) *Association between perceived inadequate staffing and musculoskeletal pain among hospital patient care workers. Int Arch Occup Environ Health; 87: 323-30.*

Koch P, Stranzinger J, Nienhaus A, Kozak A. (2015) *Musculoskeletal Symptoms and Risk of Burnout in Child Care Workers – A Cross-Sectional Study. PLOS ONE; 10: e0140980.*

Kolleck B. (2004) *Rauchen in der pflegerischen Ausbildung. Pflege; 17: 98-104.*

Kostelnik K, Heuwieser W. (2009) *Die Tiermedizin im Wandel: Nachwuchsmangel in der Nutztier-medizin. Dtsch tierärztl Wschr; 9: 412-20.*

Kozak A, Wendeler D, Schedlbauer G, Nienhaus A. (2012) *Unfälle und Berufskrankheiten bei Beschäftigten in Tierarztpraxen – Fallzahlen der Jahre 2007 bis 2011. DTBl; 9: 1230-36.*

Kung J, Chiappelli F, Cajulis OO, Avezova R, Kossan G, Chew L, Maida CA. (2010) *From Systematic Reviews to Clinical Recommendations for Evidence-Based Health Care: Validation of Revised Assessment of Multiple Systematic Reviews (R-AMSTAR) for Grading of Clinical Relevance. The Open Dentistry Journal; 4: 84-91.*

Kuorinka I, Jonsson B, Kilbom A, Vinterberg H, Biering-Sorensen F, Andersson G, Jorgensen K. (1987) *Standardised Nordic questionnaires for the analysis of musculoskeletal symptoms. Appl Ergon; 18: 233-7.*

Lang J, Ochsmann E, Kraus T, Lang JWB. (2012) *Psychosocial work stressors as antecedents of musculoskeletal problems: A systematic review and meta-analysis of stability-adjusted longitudinal studies. Soc Sci Med; 75: 1163-74.*

Lee CE, Simmonds MJ, Novy DM, Jones S. (2001) *Self-reports and clinician-measured physical function among patients with low back pain: a comparison. Arch Phys Med Rehabil; 82: 227-31.*

Lewinsohn PM, Rohde P, Seeley JR. (1998) *Major depressive disorder in older adolescents: prevalence, risk factors, and clinical implications. Clin Psychol Rev; 18: 765-94.*

Liebers F, Caffier G. (2009) *Berufsspezifische Arbeitsunfähigkeit durch Muskel-Skelett-Erkrankungen in Deutschland. F1996, Bundesanstalt für Arbeitsschutz und Arbeitsmedizin (BAuA), ed., Dortmund, Berlin, Dresden.*

Lindeman K, Kugler J, Klewer J. (2011) *Ernährungsgewohnheiten, BMI und Diätversuche von Auszubildenden in Gesundheitsfachberufen. HeilberufeScience; 2: 67-70.*

Loomans J, Weeren-Bitterling M, Weeren P, Barneveld A. (2008) *Occupational disability and job satisfaction in the equine veterinary profession: How sustainable is this 'tough job' in a changing world? Equine Vet Educ; 20: 597-607.*

Lozano-Calderon S, Anthony S, Ring D. (2008) *The quality and strength of evidence for etiology: example of carpal tunnel syndrome. J Hand Surg Am; 33: 525-38.*

Lucas M, Day L, Shirangi A, Fritschi L. (2009) *Significant injuries in Australian veterinarians and use of safety precautions. Occup Med (Lond); 59: 327-33.*

Mattioli S, Zanardi F, Baldasseroni A, Schaafsma F, Cooke RM, Mancini G, Fierro M, Santangelo C, Farioli A, Fucksia S, Curti S, Violante FS, Verbeek J. (2010) *Search strings for the study of putative occupational determinants of disease. Occup Environ Med; 67: 436-43.*

McBeth J, Jones K. (2007) *Epidemiology of chronic musculoskeletal pain. Best Pract Res Clin Rheumatol; 21: 403-25.*

McGrath BJ, Huntington AD. (2007) *The health and wellbeing of adults working in early childhood education. AJEC; 32: 33-38.*

Mediouni Z, de Roquemaurel A, Dumontier C, Becour B, Garrabe H, Roquelaure Y, Descatha A. (2014) *Is carpal tunnel syndrome related to computer exposure at work? A review and meta-analysis. J Occup Environ Med; 56: 204-8.*

Meyer M, Böttcher M, Glushanok I. (2015) *Krankheitsbedingte Fehlzeiten in der deutschen Wirtschaft im Jahr 2014. In: Fehlzeiten-Report 2015. (Bardura B, Ducki A, Schröder H, Klose J, Meyer M, ed.), Springer-Verlag: Berlin, Heidelberg, 341-538.*

Mitchell T, O'Sullivan PB, Burnett A, Straker L, Smith A, Thornton J, Rudd CJ. (2010) *Identification of modifiable personal factors that predict new-onset low back pain: a prospective study of female nursing students. Clin J Pain; 26: 275-83.*

Mitchell T, O'Sullivan PB, Smith A, Burnett AF, Straker L, Thornton J, Rudd CJ. (2009) *Biopsychosocial factors are associated with low back pain in female nursing students: a cross-sectional study. Int J Nurs Stud; 46: 678-88.*

Neumann P, Klewer J. (2010) *Das Gesundheitsverhalten von Auszubildenden im sozialpflegerischen Bereich – Eine Untersuchung an Berufsbildenden Schulen in Sachsen. Pflegewissenschaft; 12/10:672-77.*

Nienhaus A, Skudlik C, Seidler A. (2005) *Work-related accidents and occupational diseases in veterinarians and their staff. Int Arch Occup Environ Health; 78: 230-8.*

Norwood S, McAuley C, Vallina VL, Fernandez LG, McLarty JW, Goodfried G. (2000) *Mechanisms and patterns of injuries related to large animals. J Trauma; 48: 740-4.*

Nübling M, Stößel U, Hasselhorn H, Michaelis M, Hofmann F. (2005) *Methoden zur Erfassung psychischer Belastungen. Erprobung eines Messinstrumentes (COPSOQ). Wirtschaftsverlag NW: Bremerhaven.*

Nussbaum MA, Torres N. (2001) *Effects of training in modifying working methods during common patient-handling activities. Int J Ind Ergon; 27: 33-41.*

Occhionero V, Korpinen L, Gobba F. (2014) *Upper limb musculoskeletal disorders in healthcare personnel. Ergonomics; 57: 1166-91.*

Ochsmann E, Winkler R. (2009) *Übersicht arbeitsbezogener Muskelskeletterkrankungen, gegliedert nach betroffenen Regionen und Diagnose, und deren Häufigkeit in verschiedenen Tätigkeitsfeldern und Berufsgruppen, Institut für Arbeitsmedizin und Sozialmedizin (IASA), ed., http://www.dguv.de/de/Pr%C3%A4vention/Kampagnen-Veranstaltungen-und-Projekte/Pr%C3% A4ventionskampagnen/Risiko-raus!/Literatur-Report/index.jsp (Stand 28.12.2015).*

Olson MW, Li L, Solomonow M. (2004) *Flexion-relaxation response to cyclic lumbar flexion. Clinical Biomechanics; 19: 769-76.*

Olson MW, Li L, Solomonow M. (2009) *Interaction of viscoelastic tissue compliance with lumbar muscles during passive cyclic flexion-extension. J Electromyogr Kinesiol; 19: 30-8.*

OSHA, Occupational Safety and Health Administration (2009) *Guidelines for nursing homes – ergo nomics for the prevention of musculoskeletal disorders. OSHA 3182-3R 2009, https://www.osha. gov/ergonomics/guidelines/nursinghome/final_nh_guidelines. html (Stand 20.09.2015).*

Palmer KT, Harris EC, Coggon D. (2007) *Carpal tunnel syndrome and its relation to occupation: a systematic literature review. Occup Med (Lond); 57: 57-66.*

PEROSH. (2012) *OSH Evidence Methods – Clearinghouse of Systematic Reviews, Partnership for European Research in Occupational Safety and Health (PEROSH), ed., http://www.perosh.eu/research-projects/perosh-projects/occupational-safety-and-health-evidenceclearinghouse/ (Stand 19.04. 2014).*

Picavet HS, Hoeymans N. (2004) *Health related quality of life in multiple musculoskeletal diseases: SF-36 and EQ-5D in the DMC3 study. Ann Rheum Dis; 63: 723-9.*

Pieper D, Antoine SL, Mathes T, Neugebauer EA, Eikermann M. (2014) *Systematic review finds overlapping reviews were not mentioned in every other overview. J Clin Epidemiol; 67: 368-75.*

Pieper D, Buchter RB, Antoine SL, Eikermann M. (2013) *[Overviews – status quo, potentials and perspectives]. Zeitschrift für Evidenz, Fortbildung und Qualitat im Gesundheitswesen; 107: 592-6.*

Plass D, Vos T, Hornberg C, Scheidt-Nave C, Zeeb H, Krämer A. (2014) *Entwicklung der Krankheitslast in Deutschland. Dtsch Arztebl International; 111: 629-38.*

Pohjonen T, Punakallio A, Louhevaara V. (1998) *Participatory ergonomics for reducing load and strain in home care work. Int J Ind Ergon; 21: 345-52.*

Pompeii LA, Lipscomb HJ, Schoenfisch AL, Dement JM. (2009) *Musculoskeletal injuries resulting from patient handling tasks among hospital workers. Am J Ind Med; 52: 571-8.*

Purcell C, Moyle W, Evans K. (2006) *An exploration of modifiable health associated risk factors within a cohort of undergraduate nursing students. Contemp Nurse; 23: 100-10.*

Randall E, Hansen C, Gilkey D, Patil A, Bachand A, Rosecrance J, Douphrate D. (2012) *Evaluation of ergonomic risk factors among veterinary ultrasonographers.Vet Radiol Ultrasound; 53: 459-64.*

Reijula K, Rasanen K, Hamalainen M, Juntunen K, Lindbohm ML, Taskinen H, Bergbom B, Rinta-Jouppi M. (2003) *Work environment and occupational health of Finnish veterinarians. Am J IndMed; 44: 46-57.*

Reinert DF, Allen JP. (2007) *The alcohol use disorders identification test: an update of research findings. Alcohol Clin Exp Res; 31: 185-99.*

Rempel D, Evanoff B, Amadio PC, de Krom M, Franklin G, Franzblau A, Gray R, Gerr F, Hagberg M, Hales T, Katz JN, Pransky G. (1998) *Consensus criteria for the classification of carpal tunnel syndrome in epidemiologic studies. Am J Public Health; 88: 1447-51.*

Remschmidt H. (2013) *Adoleszenz – seelische Gesundheit und psychische Krankheit. Dtsch Arztebl International; 110: 423-24.*

Ribeiro DC, Aldabe D, Abbott JH, Sole G, Milosavljevic S. (2012) *Dose-response relationship between work-related cumulative postural exposure and low back pain: a systematic review. Ann Occup Hyg; 56: 684-96.*

Ribeiro DC, Sole G, Abbott JH, Milosavljevic S. (2011) *Cumulative postural exposure measured by a novel device: a preliminary study. Ergonomics; 54: 858-65.*

Roffey DM, Wai EK, Bishop P, Kwon BK, Dagenais S. (2010) *Causal assessment of awkward occupational postures and low back pain: results of a systematic review. Spine J; 10: 89-99.*

Rothgang H, Müller R, Unger R. (2012) *Themenreport „Pflege 2030" – Was ist zu erwarten – Was ist zu tun?*, Bertelsmann Stiftung, ed., *https://www.bertelsmann-stiftung.de/fileadmin/files/BSt/Publikationen/GrauePublikationen/GP_Themenreport_Pflege_2030.pdf (Stand 15.12.2015).*

Roux CH, Guillemin F, Boini S, Longuetaud F, Arnault N, Hercberg S, Briancon S. (2005) *Impact of musculoskeletal disorders on quality of life: an inception cohort study. Ann Rheum Dis; 64: 606-11.*

Rudman A, Gustavsson JP. (2012) *Burnout during nursing education predicts lower occupational preparedness and future clinical performance: a longitudinal study. Int J Nurs Stud; 49: 988-1001.*

Schwanke A, Bomball J, Schmitt S, Stöver M, Görres S. (2011) *Gesundheitsförderung und Prävention in Pflegeschulen – Ergebnisse einer Studie zur bundesweiten Vollerhebung in Pflegeschulen. Pflegewissenschaft; 4: 205-12.*

Scuffham AM, Firth EC, Stevenson MA, Legg SJ. (2010 a) *Tasks considered by veterinarians to cause them musculoskeletal discomfort, and suggested solutions. N Z Vet J; 58: 37-44.*

Scuffham AM, Legg SJ, Firth EC, Stevenson MA. (2010 b) *Prevalence and risk factors associated with musculoskeletal discomfort in New Zealand veterinarians. Appl Ergon; 41: 444-53.*

Simon M, Tackenberg P, Hasselhorn HM, Kümmerling A, Büschner A, Müller BH. (2005) *Auswertung der ersten Befragung der NEXT-Studie in Deutschland, Bergische Universität Wuppertal; Universität Witten/Herdecke, ed., http://www.next.uni-wuppertal.de/index.php?artikel-und-berichte-1 (Stand 21.05.2015).*

Singleton EK, Bienemy C, Hutchinson SW, Dellinger A, Rami JS. (2011) *A pilot study: a descriptive correlational study of factors associated with weight in college nursing students. ABNF J; 22: 89-95.*

Singleton G. (2005) *Shoulder injuries in veterinary surgeons. Vet Rec; 157: 491-2.*

Smith DR, Leggat PA, Speare R. (2009) *Musculoskeletal disorders and psychosocial risk factors among veterinarians in Queensland, Australia. Aust Vet J; 87: 260-5.*

Solomonow M. (2004) *Ligaments: a source of work-related musculoskeletal disorders. J Electromyogr Kinesiol; 14: 49-60.*

Solomonow M, Baratta RV, Banks A, Freudenberger C, Zhou BH. (2004) *Flexion–relaxation response to static lumbar flexion in males and females. Clinical Biomechanics; 18: 273-79.*

Spahn G, Wollny J, Hartmann B, Schiele R, Hofmann GO. (2012) *[Metaanalysis for the evaluation of risk factors for carpal tunnel syndrome (CTS) Part II. Occupational risk factors]. Z Orthop Unfall; 150: 516-24.*

Stroup DF, Berlin JA, Morton SC, Olkin I, Williamson GD, Rennie D, Moher D, Becker BJ, Sipe TA, Thacker SB. (2000) *Meta-analysis of observational studies in epidemiology: a proposal for reporting. Meta-analysis Of Observational Studies in Epidemiology (MOOSE) group. JAMA; 283: 2008-12.*

Timmins F, Corroon AM, Byrne G, Mooney B. (2011) *The challenge of contemporary nurse education programmes. Perceived stressors of nursing students: mental health and related lifestyle issues. J Psychiatr Ment Health Nurs; 18: 758-66.*

TK, Techniker Krankenkasse (2013) *Gesundheitsreport 2013 – Berufstätigkeit, Ausbildung und Gesundheit. https://www.tk.de/centaurus/servlet/contentblob/516416/Datei/2700/Gesundheitsreport-2013.pdf (Stand 14.12.2015).*

TK, Techniker Krankenkasse (2015) *Gesundheitsreport 2015 – Gesundheit von Studierenden. https://www.tk.de/tk/broschueren-und-mehr/studien-und-auswertungen/gesundheitsreport-2015/718618 (Stand 16.12.2015).*

Toomingas A, Nemeth G, Alfredsson L. (1995) *Self-administered examination versus conventional medical examination of the musculoskeletal system in the neck, shoulders, and upper limbs. The Stockholm MUSIC I Study Group. J Clin Epidemiol; 48: 1473-83.*

Tullar JM, Brewer S, Amick BC, Irvin E, Mahood Q, Pompeii LA, Wang A, Van Eerd D, Gimeno D, Evanoff B. (2010) *Occupational safety and health interventions to reduce musculoskeletal symptoms in the health care sector. J Occup Rehabil; 20: 199-219.*

van Rijn RM, Huisstede BM, Koes BW, Burdorf A. (2009) *Associations between work-related factors and the carpal tunnel syndrome--a systematic review. Scand J Work Environ Health; 35: 19-36.*

Videman T, Rauhala H, Asp S, Lindstrom K, Cedercreutz G, Kamppi M, Tola S, Troup JD. (1989) *Patient-handling skill, back injuries, and back pain. An intervention study in nursing. Spine (Phila Pa 1976); 14: 148-56.*

Viikari-Juntura E, Silverstein B. (1999) *Role of physical load factors in carpal tunnel syndrome. Scand J Work Environ Health; 25: 163-85.*

Violante FS, Armstrong TJ, Fiorentini C, Graziosi F, Risi A, Venturi S, Curti S, Zanardi F, Cooke RM, Bonfiglioli R, Mattioli S. (2007) *Carpal tunnel syndrome and manual work: a longitudinal study. J Occup Environ Med; 49: 1189-96.*

Wai EK, Roffey DM, Bishop P, Kwon BK, Dagenais S. (2010) *Causal assessment of occupational bending or twisting and low back pain: results of a systematic review. Spine J; 10: 76-88.*

Walton DM, Carroll LJ, Kasch H, Sterling M, Verhagen AP, Macdermid JC, Gross A, Santaguida PL, Carlesso L. (2013) *An Overview of Systematic Reviews on Prognostic Factors in Neck Pain: Results from the International Collaboration on Neck Pain (ICON) Project. Open Orthop J; 7: 494-505.*

Watson H, Whyte R, Schartau E, Jamieson E. (2006) *Survey of student nurses and midwives: smoking and alcohol use. Br J Nurs; 15: 1212-6.*

Wendeler D, Dulon M, Nienhaus A. (2015) *Unfälle und Berufskrankheiten im Jahr 2013 bei der BGW. In: Risiken und Ressourcen in Gesundheitsdienst und Wohlfahrtspflege. Band 2, (Nienhaus A, ed.), ecomed: Landsberg am Lech, 17-36.*

Whitlock EP, Lin JS, Chou R, Shekelle P, Robinson KA. (2008) *Using existing systematic reviews in complex systematic reviews. Ann Intern Med; 148: 776-82.*

Wilke HJ, Neef P, Caimi M, Hoogland T, Claes LE. (1999) *New in vivo measurements of pressures in the intervertebral disc in daily life. Spine (Phila Pa 1976); 24: 755-62.*

Yamalik N. (2007) *Musculoskeletal disorders (MSDs) and dental practice Part 2. Risk factors for dentistry, magnitude of the problem, prevention, and dental ergonomics. Int Dent J; 57: 45-54.*

Yassi A, Lockhart K. (2013) *Work-relatedness of low back pain in nursing personnel: a systematic review. Int J Occup Environ Health; 19: 223-44.*

Yip VY. (2004) *New low back pain in nurses: work activities, work stress and sedentary lifestyle. J Adv Nurs; 46: 430-40.*

You D, Smith AH, Rempel D. (2014) *Meta-analysis: association between wrist posture and carpal tunnel syndrome among workers. Safety and Health at Work; 5: 27-31.*

4 Publikationen

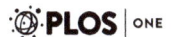

Self-Reported Musculoskeletal Disorders of the Distal Upper Extremities and the Neck in German Veterinarians: A Cross-Sectional Study

Agnessa Kozak[1]*, Grita Schedlbauer[2], Claudia Peters[1], Albert Nienhaus[1,2]

1 Institute for Health Services Research in Dermatology and Nursing, University Medical Center Hamburg-Eppendorf, Hamburg, Germany, 2 Department of Occupational Health Research, Institution for Statutory Accident Insurance and Prevention in Healthcare and Welfare, Hamburg, Germany

Abstract

Background: Veterinary work is a physically demanding profession and entails the risk of injuries and diseases of the musculoskeletal system, particularly in the upper body. The prevalence of musculoskeletal disorders (MSD), the consequences and work-related accidents in German veterinarians were investigated. Work-related and individual factors associated with MSD of upper extremities and the neck were analyzed.

Methods: In 2011, a self-reporting Standardized Nordic Questionnaire was mailed to registered veterinarians in seven federal medical associations in Germany. A total of 3174 (38.4%) veterinarians responded. Logistic regression analysis was used to determine the association between risk factors and MSD-related impairment of daily activities.

Results: MSD in the neck (66.6%) and shoulder (60.5%) were more prevalent than in the hand (34.5%) or elbow (24.5%). Normal activities were affected in 28.7% (neck), 29.5% (shoulder), 19.4% (hand) and 14% (elbow) of the respondents. MSD in the upper body occurred significantly more often in large animal practitioners. Accidents that resulted in MSD were most frequently reported in the hand/wrist (14.3%) or in the shoulder (10.8%). The majority of all accidents in the distal upper extremities were caused by animals than by other factors (19% vs. 9.2%). For each area of the body, a specific set of individual and work-related factors contributed significantly to severe MSD: Older age, gender, previous injuries, BMI, practice type, veterinary procedures such as dentistry, rectal procedures and obstetric procedures as well as high demands and personal burnout.

Conclusion: From the perspective of occupational health and safety, it seems to be necessary to improve accident prevention and to optimize the ergonomics of specific tasks. Our data suggest the need for target group-specific preventive measures that also focus on the psychological factors at work.

Citation: Kozak A, Schedlbauer G, Peters C, Nienhaus A (2014) Self-Reported Musculoskeletal Disorders of the Distal Upper Extremities and the Neck in German Veterinarians: A Cross-Sectional Study. PLoS ONE 9(2): e89362. doi:10.1371/journal.pone.0089362

Editor: Carlos M. Isales, Georgia Regents University, United States of America

Received August 13, 2013; **Accepted** January 21, 2014; **Published** February 19, 2014

Funding: The authors have no support or funding to report.

Competing Interests: The authors have declared that no competing interests exist.

* E-mail: a.kozak@uke.de

Introduction

Recent studies on professional veterinarians have demonstrated that veterinary work is physically demanding and poses an elevated risk of significant injuries [1–4]. A number of physical and psychological risk factors at work, particular in veterinary professions, have been linked to musculoskeletal disorders (MSD): static or awkward postures, repetitive or forceful tasks, animal related injuries, pressure of time, work stress, career structure or after hours duties [5–8]. Equine and bovine practitioners regularly undertake repetitive tasks, such as rectal palpation or obstetric procedures, which require lifting or exerting an upward force and/ or resisting animals' unpredictable movements [4]. Some practitioners work with one or both arms above shoulder level for over one hour daily [7]. These postures and movements may be risk factors for the development of MSD in the upper extremities in veterinarians [6,9]. Ailsby, for instance, assumed that an occupational neck- shoulder- and arm-syndrome is significantly

associated with continuous or repeated strain from repetitive and forceful motions during veterinary work (e.g. procedures such as rectal examinations or calving) [10]. Such microtrauma or minute injuries from repeatedly overusing a specific part of the body result in conditions called "Repetitive Strain Injuries" or "Cumulative Trauma Disorders" (CTD). In the literature, those conditions are summarized under the higher level term of "Work-Related Musculoskeletal Disorders of Upper Extremities" (WRMSDs-UE), which are inflammatory and degenerative disorders responsible for pain and functional impairment in tendons, muscles, joints, nerves or blood vessels [11].

Work-related accidents constitute a further health risk factor. According to the insurance data from the Statutory Accident Insurance in the Health and Welfare Services in Germany (BGW-Berufsgenossenschaft für Gesundheitsdienst und Wohlfahrtspflege) for the 5-year period (1998–2002) of all reported claims, work-related accidents accounted for 87.7% of claims in veterinary practice. Animals (66%) were the main cause of these accidents [12]. Numerous studies have shown that veterinarians are at high risk of significant acute traumatic injury (ATI) from animal contacts - predominantly in the upper extremities [2,13–15]. Large animal practitioners are most likely to suffer severe injuries [8,16]. In particular, palpation is one of the five most common causes of injuries in veterinary practitioners [13]. The risk of job-related injuries in veterinarians is higher than for other professions in the healthcare sector [12].

Therefore, working characteristics may contribute to the prevalence of MSD symptoms in veterinarians. They may suffer from work-related physical impairment or disability in functional tasks and/or the chronic or acute musculoskeletal disease. Veterinarians are more likely to report chronic work-related musculoskeletal problems if they perform clinical work [8]. According to the registration data from the German Federal Veterinary Council, 49% of the veterinarians in Germany work in clinical practice and perform tasks and procedures which can lead to MSD [17]. However, there are no available data on the prevalence of MSD in German veterinarians.

The purpose of the present study was, therefore, to examine the self-reported prevalence for MSD, the resulting physical limitations, and the frequency of injuries in the distal upper extremities and the neck. We also investigated the relationship between demographic, occupation-related risk factors (e.g. practice type, work task or previous injury) and MSD-related impairment of daily activities (severe MSD) in the relevant body regions.

Materials and Methods

Subjects

In 2011 we conducted a survey of registered veterinarians in seven federal states in Germany (medical associations in Baden-Württemberg, Bavaria, Berlin, Brandenburg, Lower Saxony, Schleswig-Holstein, and Westphalia-Lippe). According to the registration data from the German Federal Veterinary Council, there were no statistically significant differences between responders and non-responders with respect to gender and age distribution [17]. None of the seven medical associations of the federal states in the study was overrepresented. Thus, the sample can be considered as representative.

Measurement

We measured the presence and severity of MSD during the preceding 12 months with the Standardized Nordic Questionnaire [18]. This instrument has been applied to various occupational groups to evaluate musculoskeletal problems. An anatomical sketch of labeled body regions allowed the respondents to clearly identify body areas affected by MSD. A dichotomous yes/no answer indicated whether the participants had suffered any symptoms in the queried body area during the preceding 12 months. To assess the severity, the following question was asked: *"What is the total length of time that [neck] trouble has prevented you from doing your normal work (at home or away from home) during the last 12-months?"*. Possible replies to this question were: (1) *"the discomfort was not too severe"*; (2) *"1 to 7 days"*; (3) *"8 to 30 days"* or (4) *"more than 30 days"*. We aimed to distinguish participants who felt a certain discomfort but did not experience longer lasting restrictions in work and daily life from those who were restricted for at least one week in the past 12 months. Participants who replied with *"the discomfort was not too severe"* were allocated to the non-affected group. For each queried body area, we also asked the participants whether these symptoms were caused by a work-related injury during their professional life. Work-related injuries were differen-

tiated into animal-related and other-related injuries during working hours (e.g. falls, motor vehicle accidents). The participants were asked to provide their demographic data (age and gender), anthropometric measures (height and weight), dominant hand, current job status (full-time or part-time), the type of practice (small, mixed or large animal), length of work experience, number of hours worked per week and whether they were involved in sports activities or not. We calculated the body mass index (BMI) and categorized it into normal weight (BMI<25), overweight (25–30), and obese (>30).

The veterinarians were asked to estimate the number (0; <600; 600–2400; 2400–6000; 6000–12,000; >12,000) of examinations and procedures they performed annually. The detailed list of veterinary procedures was adopted from Scuffham et al. and translated into German [4]. The following procedures were queried: (1) obstetric procedures, (2) rectal palpations, (3) inseminations, (4) vaginal examinations, (5) animal handling/lifting, (6) blood sampling, (7) vaccinations, (8) dehorning/velveting, (9) foot trimming, (10) lameness examinations, (11) necropsies, (12) ultrasonography, (13) radiography, (14) endoscopies, (15) dental procedures, (16) surgery lasting <1 hour, and (17) surgery lasting >1 hour. For the analysis, we summarized the number of procedures into three categories (0 or not specified; < 600; ≥600).

Quantitative job demands were measured by a five-point Likert scale from the Copenhagen Psychosocial Questionnaire (COP-SOQ) [19]. This scale measures the amount of work that has to be done in a particular time (e.g. intensive and extensive job demands). The frequency of typical load factors at work were measured with four questions (1. *"Do you have enough time for your work tasks?"*; 2. *"Do you have to do overtime?"*; 3. *"Is your work unevenly distributed so it piles up?"*; 4. *"Do you have to work very fast?"*). The Cronbach's Alpha value was acceptable ($\alpha = .65$). To capture the psychological condition of the veterinarians, the 'personal burnout' subscale from the Copenhagen Burnout Inventory (CBI) was applied. This scale contains six items on general symptoms of exhaustion and is defined as "the degree of physical and psychological fatigue and exhaustion experienced by the person". This five-point Likert scale ($\alpha = .87$) shows good internal consistency [20]. Both scales were transformed into a theoretical range, extending from 0 (never/almost never) to 100 (always) points. This transformation is a standardized procedure and conforms to the German validation study. If at least half of the single items had valid answers, scale scores were computed as the average of the values [21]. For the logistic regression models, we summarized the original scales into tertiles and defined them as low, medium or high. The final questionnaire was pre-tested on ten veterinarians to remove inconsistencies, detect unclear wording and to complement missing aspects.

Ethics Statement

Each questionnaire included an informative letter which clarifies the free participation and anonymity of this study. We did not ask for the written consent of the participants. The voluntary participation was deemed as informed consent. The study protocol was approved by the Hamburg Medical Council Ethics Commission (# PV3839).

Statistical Analysis

Descriptive statistics were used to describe the study sample and to estimate the prevalence of musculoskeletal disorders (MSD), the disorder severity (activities affected) and accident prevalence in the upper extremities and neck. Differences in MSD prevalence were examined using Pearson's chi-square test for categorical variables.

For collinearity analysis, we scanned the Spearman correlation matrix to avoid multicollinearity or redundancy between independent variables (e.g. job tasks). Spearman's correlation coefficients of $\rho \geq 0.6$ were considered as problematic, as they introduce a substantial bias into the estimation of the logistic regression models [22]. Thus, the variable 'job experience' was removed from the analysis, as this strongly correlated with age ($\rho = 0.8$). We found that rectal palpations were frequently mentioned as a risk factor for CTD or ATI in the upper extremities [3,6,13]. As the predictor variables foot trimming, dehorning/velveting, vaginal examinations, and inseminations showed significant moderate correlations with rectal palpations ($\rho \geq 0.6$), we decided to remove these from further analysis. Univariate logistic regressions were calculated to identify associations between severe MSD in the previous 12 months and individual, work-related and psychosocial factors in the respective body parts. As we performed a number of tests, we set the alpha level at p<0.01, in order to lower the probability of type I errors. Predictor variables which significantly affected the rate of MSD severity were selected for multivariate modeling. However, the demographic variables age and gender were included in each tested model, whether or not they had a significant influence in the univariate analysis. Backward stepwise multivariate logistic regression analyses were performed to develop a final explanatory model for each body part. The likelihood ratio statistic was used for variable entry (p<0.05) and removal (p<0.1). Analyses were performed with SPSS Version 17.0.

Results

Study Population

A total of 3174 veterinarians responded to the self-administered questionnaire (response rate 38.4%). Complete information was provided by 3051 subjects (96% of the responses). Table 1 describes the study population. The mean age of the participants was 47.6 (± 10) years, with an average of 18.0 (± 10.2) years of job experience in veterinary practice. Of the 3051 participants in the survey, the majority (97.1%) worked in a clinical practice and 82% were self employed. Most study participants were small animal practitioners (48.6%). The proportion of women working in small animal practices was significantly higher (75.2%) than in mixed (38.9%) and large (31.8%) animal practices (p<0.001) and vice versa (25% of men worked in small, 61% in mixed and 68% in large animal practices). Thus, there was a gender difference in the tasks performed in veterinary practice. Male practitioners significantly more often performed tasks related to a job profile in mixed and large animal practices (e.g. rectal palpations or obstetric procedures). Table 2 shows relevant veterinary tasks which significantly correlated with practice type (Spearman's correlation of at least $\rho = 0.2$). The tasks are ranked according to their relevance (high to low correlation). Large and mixed animal practitioners more often performed foot trimming, rectal palpations, inseminations, dehorning/velveting, vaginal examinations and obstetric procedures. Small animal practitioners, however, more often performed x-rays, handling and lifting, dental procedures and surgeries.

Prevalence of MSD Symptoms

Of those affected, a quarter reported MSD trouble in one body site, 56% reported two to three body sites, and 8% experienced MSD in four queried body sites. The prevalence of MSD by body site is given in Table 3, stratified by gender and practice type. The prevalences of the MSD symptoms in the upper extremities in the preceding 12 months differed considerably; the highest prevalences were observed in the neck (66.6%) and shoulder region (60.5%).

Table 1. Characteristics of the study population.

Variables		N = 3051 (%)
Sex	Female	1657 (54.3)
	Male	1394 (45.7)
Age*	<30	105 (3.4)
	30–39	561 (18.4)
	40–49	1081 (35.4)
	>50	1304 (42.7)
	>50	1304 (42.7)
BMI	<25	1733 (56.8)
	25–30	1050 (34.4)
	>30	268 (8.8)
Job experience**	<10	693 (22.7)
	10–19	1003 (32.9)
	20–29	936 (30.7)
	>30	419 (13.7)
Practice type	Small	1483 (48.6)
	Mixed	614 (20.1)
	Large	954 (31.3)
Working h/week	>35 h	2471 (81.0)
	15–34 h	465 (15.2)
	<15 h	115 (3.8)
Work setting	Practice	2963 (97.1)
	Industry	57 (1.9)
	University/ Administration	24 (0.8)
	Other	7 (0.2)

Note. *Age: mean 47.6 (SD±10) years; **Job experience: mean 18.0 (SD±10.2) years.
doi:10.1371/journal.pone.0089362.t001

MSD in the hand (34.5%) and elbow (24.5%) were less frequently reported. Neck symptoms were more likely to be reported by female veterinarians (p<0.001). Male veterinarians, however, significantly more often reported symptoms in the elbow (p< 0.001). A significantly higher proportion of large animal practitioners reported MSD in the distal upper extremities than did practitioners in mixed and small practices (p<0.001).

Severe MSD (Activities Affected)

Correspondingly, the perceived physical disability in functional tasks (severe MSD) during the preceding 12 months was highest in the neck (28.7%) and shoulder (29.5%), and lowest in the hand/wrist (19.4%) and elbow (14%). Women showed higher MSD severity in the neck (p<0.001) and also in hand/wrist (p<0.01), while men reported significantly higher severe MSD in the elbow region (p<0.001). The proportion of severe MSD in the upper distal extremities increased significantly with the size of the treated animals (Table 3).

Reported Accidents

Work-related accidents that resulted in MSD complaints were most frequently reported in the hand/wrist (14.3%) and shoulder (10.8%); the least reported injuries were in the neck (6.6%) and elbow region (5.5%). Except for the neck, more accidents in the upper extremities were caused by animals than by other factors

Table 2. The frequency of veterinary tasks performed annually, stratified by practice type.

Practice type	Small (%)			Mixed (%)			Large (%)		
Veterinary tasks	0	<600	600–2400	0	<600	600–2400	0	<600	600–2400
Foot trimming	77.8	6.4	1.2	12.8	31.9	25.3	9.5	61.7	73.5
Rectal palpation	81.8	60.7	6.3	9.8	19.7	29.6	8.4	19.6	64.1
Insemination	66.7	12.8	1.3	16.0	28.1	31.2	17.3	59.1	67.4
Dehorning/velveting	65.2	3.7	13.5	15.7	32.7	18.9	19.1	63.7	67.6
Vaginal examination	72.6	41.5	8.9	13.0	22.9	27.5	14.3	35.5	63.6
Radiography	22.4	55.2	69.7	20.0	22.3	15.1	57.6	22.5	15.1
Obstetric procedure	74.5	36.1	22.1	10.9	25.4	14.7	14.6	38.6	63.2
Handling/lifting	39.8	30.4	59.2	14.2	21.1	20.1	46.0	48.5	20.7
Dental procedure	22.4	54.7	57.7	11.8	22.9	18.6	65.8	22.4	23.7
Surgery lasting <1	40.7	44.9	67.2	22.7	19.8	20.2	36.6	35.4	12.6
Surgery lasting >1	37.2	50.2	68.4	18.7	20.8	17.2	44.1	29.0	14.4

Note. The differences between practice types were significant (p<0.05) for all procedures.
doi:10.1371/journal.pone.0089362.t002

(19% vs. 9.2%). Male practitioners were more likely to report injuries in the neck (11.4% vs. 6.5%), shoulders (23.4% vs. 10.1%), elbows (20.7% vs. 12.6%), and hand/wrist (36.5% vs. 30.1%) than female practitioners. Except for the elbow, the accident rate increases proportionally (p<0.05) with the age of the practitioners. Large and mixed animal practitioners were more likely to report accidents in the neck (14%, 13% and 3.6%, respectively), shoulder (24.2%, 25% and 6.4%, respectively) and elbow (23.2%, 17.8% and 10.4%, respectively, p<0.001) than small animal practitioners. No significant differences were found for accidents in the hand/wrist (35.2%, 36.2% and 29.6%, respectively; no Table).

Risk Factors for Severe MSD

Logistic regression analysis was used to identify factors influencing the risk of MSD causing restricted movements and restricted daily activities during the preceding 12 months. The analysis was performed separately for individual regions of the upper extremities; the results are shown in Tables 4, 5, 6, 7. As some predictor variables are the same for different body regions, we describe the results together.

Veterinarians of 40 years and older run a higher risk of having physical disability in the neck (OR 2.0, 95% CI 1.2–3.3), shoulder (OR 2.1, 95% CI 1.2–2.0), elbow (>40 years: OR 11.6, 95% CI 2.8–47.9; >50 years: 13.4, 95% CI 3.2–55.9), and hand (OR 2.1 95% CI 1.0–4.1) than their younger colleagues. Severe MSD of the hand was found more often in women (OR 1.6, 95% CI 1.2–2.1), whereas female veterinarians complained of MSD in the elbow less often than their male colleagues (OR 0.7, 95% CI 0.6–0.9). Furthermore, previous accidents increased the risk of physical impairment in neck (OR 2.1, 95% CI 1.6–2.9), shoulder (OR 1.6, 95% CI 1.2–2.0), and hand (OR 1.5, 95% CI 1.2–1.9). Veterinarians with a BMI of 25–30 had 1.3 (95% CI 1.1–1.7) times the odds of MSD severity in the elbow, compared with those who had normal BMI. Veterinarians in mixed (OR 1.5, 95% CI 1.1–2.1) and large (OR 1.9, 95% CI 1.4–2.7) practices showed a higher risk for severe MSD in the elbow than small animal practitioners.

Table 3. Twelve month MSD prevalence and severe MSD (activities affected) of the upper body, stratified by gender and practice type.

Body region		Neck		Shoulder		Elbow		Hand/Wrist	
12-month prevalence		MSD experience	Severe MSD	MSD experience	Severe MSD	MSD experience	Severe MSD	MSD experience	Severe MSD
		n (%)	n (%)	n (%)	n (%)	n (%)	n (%)	n (%)	n (%)
Female n = 1657	Total	1240 (74.8)	527 (31.8)	995 (60.0)	466 (28.1)	336 (20.3)	198 (11.9)	592 (35.7)	350 (21.1)
	Small n = 1115	839 (75.2)	356 (31.9)	653 (58.6)	293 (26.3)	196 (17.6)	116 (10.4)	360 (32.3)	219 (19.6)
	Mixed n = 239	172 (72.0)	78 (32.6)	149 (62.3)	75 (31.4)	54 (22.6)	31 (13.0)	96 (40.2)	55 (23.0)
	Large n = 303	229 (75.6)	93 (30.7)	193 (63.7)	98 (32.3)	86 (28.4)	51 (16.8)	136 (44.9)	76 (25.1)
Male n = 1394	Total	793 (56.9)	348 (25.0)	851 (61.0)	433 (31.1)	411 (29.5)	230 (16.5)	460 (33.0)	242 (17.4)
	Small n = 368	211 (57.3)	82 (22.3)	183 (49.7)	79 (21.5)	77 (20.9)	30 (8.2)	84 (22.8)	37 (10.1)
	Mixed n = 375	217 (57.9)	96 (25.6)	236 (62.9)	114 (30.4)	112 (29.9)	67 (17.9)	123 (32.8)	69 (18.4)
	Large n = 651	365 (56.1)	170 (26.1)	432 (66.4)	240 (36.9)	222 (34.1)	133 (20.4)	253 (38.9)	136 (20.9)
Total N = 3051		2033 (66.6)	875 (28.7)	1846 (60.5)	899 (29.5)	747 (24.5)	428 (14.0)	1052 (34.5)	592 (19.4)

doi:10.1371/journal.pone.0089362.t003

Table 4. Multivariate analysis of severe MSD in the neck.

Variables		%	Crude OR (95%CI)	Adjusted OR[†] (95%CI)
Age (years)	<30	21.9	1	1
	30–39	31.0	1.6 (0.9–2.6)	1.5 (0.9–2.6)
	40–49	29.0	1.5 (0.9–2.4)	1.6 (1.0–2.7)
	>50	27.9	1.4 (0.9–2.2)	2.0 (1.2–3.3)**
Accidents	No	35.3	1	1
	Yes	55.5	2.3 (1.7–3.1)	2.1 (1.6–2.9)**
Dental procedures	0 or n/s	26.8	1	1
	<600	28.2	1.1 (0.9–1.3)	1.0 (0.8–1.3)
	≥600	34.3	1.4 (1.1–1.9)	1.4 (1.0–1.9)*
Quantitative demands	Low	18.4	1	1
	Medium	25.7	1.5 (1.2–2.0)	1.3 (1.0–1.8)
	High	36.7	2.6 (1.9–3.4)	1.7 (1.2–2.4)**
Personal Burnout	Low	13.6	1	1
	Medium	31.6	2.9 (2.4–3.6)	2.1 (1.7–2.7)**
	High	50.8	6.6 (5.1–8.6)	4.3 (3.2–5.8)**

Note. *p<0.05; **p<0.01. [†]Gender had no effect in the final model.
doi:10.1371/journal.pone.0089362.t004

Veterinarians who frequently performed dental procedures (≥ 600 per year) were at higher risk of being affected by MSD in the neck region (OR 1.4, 95% CI 1.0–1.9), compared to those who less often or hardly ever performed such tasks. Work-related risk factors for MSD in the shoulder increased significantly with the number of annual obstetric procedures (≥600 per year: OR 2.1, 95% CI 1.2–3.5). On the contrary, veterinarians who performed up to 600 radiological examinations per year less often reported severe MSD in the shoulder (OR 0.8, 95% CI 0.6–1.0). The risk of severe MSD in the elbows was associated with frequent rectal palpations (≥600 per year: OR 1.4, 95% CI 1.0–2.0). High quantitative demands and elevated levels of personal burnout showed consistent association with perceived severe MSD severity in all queried body regions, compared with those who less often reported pressure of time due to heavy workload and emotional exhaustion (Tables 4, 5, 6, 7).

Table 5. Multivariate analysis of severe MSD in the shoulder.

Variables		%	Crude OR (95%CI)	Adjusted OR[†] (95%CI)
Age (years)	<30	21.0	1	1
	30–39	23.9	1.2 (0.7–2.0)	1.3 (0.8–2.3)
	40–49	29.6	1.6 (1.0–2.6)	2.1 (1.2–3.6)**
	>50	32.4	1.8 (1.1–2.9)	2.1 (1.2–2.0)**
Accidents	No	42.1	1	1
	Yes	55.5	1.7 (1.3–2.2)	1.6 (1.2–2.0)**
Obstetrics	0 or n/s	22.3	1	1
	<600	32.7	1.7 (1.4–2.0)	1.4 (1.2–1.8)**
	≥600	42.1	2.5 (1.6–3.9)	2.1 (1.2–3.5)**
Radiography	0 or n/s	33.1	1	1
	<600	26.1	0.7 (0.6–0.8)	0.8 (0.6–1.0)*
	≥600	32.3	1.0 (0.8–1.2)	1.2 (0.9–1.4)
Quantitative demands	Low	16.8	1	1
	Medium	27.1	1.8 (1.4–2.5)	1.7 (1.2–2.4)**
	High	37.3	3.0 (2.2–4.0)	2.0 (1.4–2.9)**
Personal Burnout	Low	18.5	1	1
	Medium	31.5	2.0 (1.7–2.5)	2.0 (1.6–2.5)**
	High	46.0	3.8 (2.9–4.8)	3.7 (2.7–5.1)**

Note. *p<0.05; **p<0.01. [†]Gender, BMI, practice type, lameness examinations, and rectal palpations had no effect in the final model.
doi:10.1371/journal.pone.0089362.t005

Table 6. Multivariate analysis of severe MSD in the elbow.

Variables		%	Crude OR (95%CI)	Adjusted OR[†] (95%CI)
Gender	Male	16.5	1	1
	Female	11.9	0.7 (0.6–0.8)	0.7 (0.6–0.9)*
Age (years)	<30	1.9	1	1
	30–39	6.6	3.6 (0.9–15.3)	3.8 (0.9–16.2)
	40–49	15.3	9.3 (2.3–37.9)	11.6 (2.8–47.9)**
	>50	17.2	10.7 (2.6–43.6)	13.4 (3.2–55.9)**
BMI (kg/m^2)	<25	11.3	1	1
	25–30	17.6	1.7 (1.3–2.1)	1.3 (1.1–1.7)*
	>30	17.5	1.7 (1.2–2.4)	1.4 (0.9–1.9)
Practice type	Small	9.8	1	1
	Mixed	16.0	1.7 (1.3–2.3)	1.5 (1.1–2.1)*
	Large	19.3	2.2 (1.7–2.8)	1.9 (1.4–2.7)**
Rectal palpations	0 or n/s	10.4	1	1
	<600	11.6	1.2 (0.9–1.5)	1.0 (0.7–1.3)
	≥600	19.9	2.2 (1.7–2.9)	1.4 (1.0–2.0)*
Quantitative demands	Low	7.6	1	1
	Medium	12.5	1.7 (1.2–2.6)	1.5 (0.9–2.2)
	High	18.5	2.8 (1.8–4.2)	2.0 (1.3–3.2)**
Personal Burnout	Low	9.4	1	1
	Medium	15.4	1.8 (1.4–2.3)	1.8 (1.4–2.4)**
	High	19.1	2.3 (1.6–3.1)	2.3 (1.6–3.3)**

Note. *p<0.05; **p<0.01. [†]obstetric procedures, radiography had no effect in the final model.
doi:10.1371/journal.pone.0089362.t006

Table 7. Multivariate analysis of severe MSD in the hand/wrist.

Variables		%	Crude OR (95%CI)	Adjusted OR[†] (95%CI)
Gender	Male	17.4	1	1
	Female	21.1	1.3 (1.1–1.5)	1.6 (1.2–2.1)**
Age (years)	<30	14.3	1	1
	30–39	16.9	1.2 (0.7–2.2)	1.1 (0.6–2.3)
	40–49	17.4	1.3 (0.7–2.2)	1.4 (0.7–2.9)
	>50	22.5	1.7 (1.0–3.1)	2.1 (1.0–4.1)*
Accidents	No	41.2	1	1
	Yes	52.0	1.5 (1.2–1.9)	1.5 (1.2–1.9)**
Rectal palpations	0 or n/s	18.0	1	1
	<600	16.6	0.9 (0.7–1.1)	0.8 (0.6–1.1)
	≥600	23.7	1.4 (1.1–1.8)	1.2 (0.9–1.7)
Quantitative demands	Low	17.3	1	1
	Medium	19.2	1.1 (0.9–1.4)	1.4 (0.9–2.1)
	High	27.5	1.8 (1.3–2.5)	1.8 (1.2–2.8)**
Personal Burnout	Low	13.0	1	1
	Medium	20.9	1.8 (1.4–2.2)	1.6 (1.2–2.1)**
	High	27.6	2.5 (1.9–3.4)	1.9 (1.4–2.9)**

Note. *p<0.05; **p<0.01. [†]practice type and radiography had no effect in the final model.
doi:10.1371/journal.pone.0089362.t007

Discussion

To our knowledge, this is the first large scale self-reported survey of German veterinarians which examines MSD prevalence, its severity as manifested in restricted daily activities, and work-related accidents. In line with international literature, this study showed that MSD in the distal upper extremities and the neck was frequent in this professional group. The type of veterinary practice was related to MSD prevalence and severity. In addition, work-related accidents that resulted in MSD symptoms were most frequently reported in the hand/wrist and shoulder region. The majority of all injuries in the distal upper extremities were caused by animals. Working and individual characteristics were shown to attribute to MSD severity in the upper body.

Two studies from Australia and New Zealand using the same measuring instrument also found the highest 12-month symptoms prevalence in the neck (57%–58%) and shoulder (52%–59%), followed by the hand (32%–52%) and elbow (17%–29%) [4]. However, a Dutch veterinary cohort reported symptoms in the upper extremities significantly less often (37%, 38%, 14% and 11%, respectively) [23]. The 12-month prevalence in our study was much higher than the values found in comparable professions in international studies (e.g. nurses, farmers, physicians or chiropodists) [24–27]. The prevalence values are also much higher than those found in surveys with other employees. According to a survey in Germany, about 46% of subjects complained of pain in the neck and shoulder region. About 20% of employees had pain in the arms and hands [28]. In agreement with the findings of previous studies, multiple anatomical regions were often affected [1,4,7]. In their large-scale survey in France, Roquelaure et al. found that MSD symptoms of the upper limbs often overlapped two anatomical body regions, particularly the neck and shoulder regions [29]. The type of veterinary practice was related to MSD prevalence and severity, which is in line with the results from other studies on hazards and disorders [3,4,6,8,16,30]. Practitioners in mixed and large animal practices much more frequently reported MSD in the upper body. In a study from the Netherlands, problems related to the musculoskeletal system of the upper body were by far the most important disorders in equine practitioners [1]. We found higher MSD prevalences for women in the neck and hand/wrist and for men in the elbow. Studies on general and working populations have reported higher MSD prevalences in woman than in men. Besides, women more often reported pain at more than one body site [31,32].

A small but considerable number of participants had MSD symptoms which were serious enough to affect their daily activities. From the occupational perspective, this is of critical importance, as it probably affects the veterinarians' quality of life and may also lead to changes in professional activities. This in turn may cause a loss in productivity and/or loss of earnings. The participants of the aforementioned studies less frequently reported that MSD prevented them from carrying out their daily activities than those in our study [4,5]. To some extent, this may be attributed to the differences in the definition of items used. In this context, it should be pointed out that studies with additional diagnostic measuring procedures observed significantly lower values of MSD in the neck-shoulder region and lower back [33–35]. In a study on bovine practitioners, the self reported pathological findings of CTD were also lower than the prevalence of any musculoskeletal problem [6]. Thus, it would be desirable to verify the present results through further investigations with objective procedures. However, by choosing severe MSD as an outcome measure, we aimed to identify those cases with MSD complaints which were serious enough to prevent them from performing their daily activities for at least seven days in the previous 12 months.

The present study demonstrates that hand/wrist and shoulder are frequently affected by work-related accidents. A German study which analyzed the occupational records (accidents and diseases) of veterinary staff over a 5-year period found that the hand (48.3%) and arm (17.3%) were the most affected anatomical locations. They also found that veterinarians and their staff had a 2.9-fold higher risk of injuries than general practitioners [12]. In terms of species-specific injury mechanism, our results are in keeping with previous studies, which report that work-related accidents were most frequent in large animal practices and that the upper extremities were most frequently affected [3,8,16,30]. Langley and Hunter analyzed data from the US Department of Labor on human workplace fatalities associated with animals for the years 1992–1997. They found that large animals (cattle and horses) were primarily responsible for the majority of fatal events among workers. Men and elderly workers were at greater risk of mortality [36]. This is similar to our findings; male and elderly veterinarians significantly more often reported work-related injuries. This is probably because male practitioners more frequently worked with large animals, which exposed them to greater risk of major injuries. However, the results with respect to gender were inconsistent. Some studies on injuries reported a greater risk for men [7,8], while others found that women were more often affected [3,30,37]. Some authors have argued that women are at greater risk due to their small size and limited physical strength [3,37]. In contrast to our results, previous findings showed that increasing years of experience were associated with decreasing injury-related events [13,30]. This might be explained by the higher proportion of elderly veterinarians in our study. However our results on accidents were limited, because we did not differentiate the origin and severity of the accidents in detail.

Our findings demonstrate that for each part of the body a specific set of personal and work-related factors contribute significantly to severe MSD. Older age, gender, previous injuries, BMI, practice type, veterinary procedures such as dentistry, rectal palpation, obstetrics as well as quantitatively high demands and personal burnout increased the likelihood of severe MSD in the upper extremities and the neck. Older veterinarians more often reported severe MSD in all queried body parts than their younger colleagues. The age effect described in the present study on MSD is confirmed by other studies with veterinarians [4,38]. For ageing workers, a progressive decline in physical work capacity, characterized by diminished muscular capacity, has been reported – especially for physically demanding occupations [39]. In general, the MSD are likely to become more prevalent in the veterinary profession as the working population ages and a shortage of young professionals is to be expected, especially in the large animal practices [40]. With respect to gender, women showed a higher risk of severe MSD in the hand and men in the elbow. This could be due to different mechanical patterns of procedures undertaken and/or differences in physique. According to Berry et al., women and men reported different procedures which caused them CTD; men more often reported rectal palpation and calving manipulation while women reported holding instruments, computer work and other causes [3]. The activity profile that causes MSD is greatly dependent on the type of practice. Scuffham et al. asked veterinarians about routine activities that triggered MSD in them. Large and mixed animal veterinarians mostly considered that rectal examinations, obstetric treatment, ultrasound examinations and diagnostic testing on the hoof and lameness were stressful activities. On the other hand, small animal veterinarians found that lifting and transporting animals was stressful, together with surgeries [41]. In a subsequent study, it was shown that large animal veterinarians and veterinarians who only worked with horses exhibit the greatest prevalence of MSD periods in comparison to veterinarians in other practices or organizations [4]. Cattell found that 71% of CTD and 31% of ATI to veterinarians in large animal practices were related to rectal examinations [6]. Thus, in view of the activity profile, it is plausible in the present study that mixed and large animal veterinarians, who also performed rectal palpations, significantly more often reported symptoms in the elbows. Symptoms in the shoulders correlate with frequent vaginal investigations, whereby the type of practice played a lesser role in the corresponding analysis model. In addition, dental examinations correlated with symptoms in the neck. It is known that this region is susceptible for MSD - not only for human dentists, but also for veterinarians specializing in dentistry [42,43].

Furthermore, participants in our study who reported previous work-related accidents had a higher chance of developing MSD in the neck, shoulder and hand/wrist. These results were also supported by Randall et al., who examined ergonomic risk factors among veterinary sonographers [38]. Thus, trauma acquired at work may have serious long-term consequences. Precautionary measures, such as training in body posture and handling animals, are of increasing importance in this profession. Ergonomics of the work environment can also be considered to decrease the incidence of injuries to the neck (e.g. for practitioners that have higher incidence of neck pathology).

In the current study, quantitative demands and personal burnout were associated with significant increases in MSD in all queried body regions. The association between psychosocial factors and MSD is well documented [44]. The relationship between MSD period prevalence and quantitative demands caused by time pressure and work overload was consistent with two recent studies from Australia and New Zealand [4,5]. The assumption is that a mismatch of the amount of work and the time available to do it may lead to stress [45]. Thus, MSD is not only triggered by physical factors (e.g. lifting, repetitive tasks), but also by emotional and psychosocial demands. For instance, Loomans et al. found an intermediate correlation in veterinarians between emotional work load and MSD of the lower body [1]. In addition, psychosocial stress in the veterinary setting is also associated with increased consumption of alcohol, tobacco and medication [46]. For these reasons, it is strongly recommended that preventive measures should be implemented to sustain and improve not only the physical but also the psychological well-being of veterinarians. However, we cannot rule out the possibility of reverse causation. Although the cross-sectional design is sufficient for making initial associations, it is ineligible to derive causal relationships.

Strengths and Limitations

Our study includes a large number of participants and is one of the most extensive international studies of veterinarians. The response rate of 38.4% corresponds well with the average response rate of 38.5% in other studies with veterinarians [4]. By using registration data, the sample size can be considered representative with respect to gender and age. The use of a common standardized questionnaire enables us to compare these results with other studies among veterinarians and other occupational groups. However, some limitations should be pointed out. The retrospective data collection of exposure and complaints is susceptible to recall bias, because of the potential for misreporting the number of veterinary procedures and MSD related events in the preceding 12 months. Our study, like others, was limited by

the inability to survey the non-respondents in depth due to methodological and organizational issues. We cannot rule out the possibility that veterinarians who suffered from MSD had greater motivation to participate in the study than those who were not affected, so that we were prone to overestimate the MSD burden in this occupational group. In addition, a healthy worker effect might potentially have resulted in minor underestimation of MSD, as some veterinarians might previously have left their occupation or remained on sick leave due to MSD or other diseases. The results may have been influenced by other potential work-related factors which were not considered when collecting data, in particular, insufficient recreation time, career structure, client interaction, perceived peer support, use of auxiliary devices or specific work activities (e.g. working in cold environments or working postures) [4,5]. This lack of data limits the ability to broadly explore the association between work-related factors and severe MSD in the upper extremities and the neck. A further limitation consists in the redundant predictors. As some veterinary procedures correlated highly with each other, we omitted a few explanatory variables in the multivariate models. The omission of the variables may limit the explanatory power of the model. However, we did not observe significant changes in the R-squared values of the analyzed models when we removed these factors. In general, causal relationships between variables cannot be derived in cross-sectional studies, although these allow us to quantify the magnitude of MSD prevalence and to identify initial associations. In order to establish causal explanations for MSD, a longitudinal study will be required, which has not yet been performed in this occupational group.

Conclusions

Our study contributes to the available evidence on the MSD and shows that these disorders are highly prevalent in the upper body of German veterinarians. The overall prevalence appears to be similar to that found in other international studies. From the perspective of occupational health and safety, it seems to be necessary to improve accident prevention and to optimize the ergonomics of specific tasks. In order to prevent MSD in the upper body, our data suggest the need for target group-specific (e.g. gender and practice type) preventive measures that also focus on the psychological factors at work. As a consequence of demographic changes, employees are remaining in their professions for longer. In particular, this applies to independent veterinarians in Germany, which emphasized the importance of preventive measures. Veterinary associations and organizations should provide their members with adequate training and information, so that they can work safely with animals and equipment. Preventive measures should be incorporated into the curriculum and explain to future veterinarians about the permanent and seasonal challenges in the individual veterinary practices and the related activities. Further research work must concentrate on the long-term consequences of veterinary work for the musculoskeletal system. The resulting knowledge could, for example, provide evidence-based aids for decision when determining and evaluating exposure in occupational diseases.

Acknowledgments

The authors would like to thank the German Federal Chamber of Veterinary Surgeons for their cooperation and support. We specifically acknowledge the Veterinary Medical Associations from Berlin, Brandenburg, Baden-Württemberg Lower Saxony, Bavaria, Westphalia-Lippe, and Schleswig-Holstein for the provision of addresses and/or consignment of the questionnaires. We thank all veterinarians for their substantial participation in the study.

Author Contributions

Conceived and designed the experiments: AK GS AN. Performed the experiments: AK GS CP AN. Analyzed the data: AK GS CP AN. Wrote the paper: AK GS CP AN.

References

1. Loomans JBA, Weeren-Bitterling MS, Weeren PR, Barneveld A (2008) Occupational disability and job satisfaction in the equine veterinary profession: How sustainable is this "tough job" in a changing world? Equine Vet Educ 20: 597–607.
2. Lucas M, Day L, Shirangi A, Fritschi L (2009) Significant injuries in Australian veterinarians and use of safety precautions. Occup Med Oxf Engl 59: 327–333. doi:10.1093/occmed/kqp070.
3. Berry SL, Susitaival P, Ahmadi A, Schenker MB (2012) Cumulative trauma disorders among California veterinarians. Am J Ind Med 55: 855–861. doi:10.1002/ajim.22076.
4. Scuffham AM, Legg SJ, Firth EC, Stevenson MA (2010) Prevalence and risk factors associated with musculoskeletal discomfort in New Zealand veterinarians. Appl Ergon 41: 444–453. doi:10.1016/j.apergo.2009.09.009.
5. Smith D, Leggat P, Speare R (2009) Musculoskeletal disorders and psychosocial risk factors among veterinarians in Queensland, Australia. Aust Vet J 87: 260–265. doi:10.1111/j.1751-0813.2009.00435.x.
6. Cattell MB (2000) Rectal palpation associated cumulative trauma disorders and acute traumatic injury affecting bovine practitioners. Bov Pr 34: 1–5.
7. Reijula K, Räsänen K, Hämäläinen M, Juntunen K, Lindbohm M-L, et al. (2003) Work environment and occupational health of Finnish veterinarians. Am J Ind Med 44: 46–57. doi:10.1002/ajim.10228.
8. Fritschi L, Day L, Shirangi A, Robertson I, Lucas M, et al. (2006) Injury in Australian veterinarians. Occup Med 56: 199–203. doi:10.1093/occmed/kqj037.
9. Singleton G (2005) Shoulder injuries in veterinary surgeons. Vet Rec 157: 491–492.
10. Ailsby RL (1996) Occupational arm, shoulder, and neck syndrome affecting large animal veterinarians. Can Vet J 37: 411.
11. Aptel M, Aublet-Cuvelier A, Claude Cnockaert J (2002) Work-related musculoskeletal disorders of the upper limb. Joint Bone Spine 69: 546–555. doi:10.1016/S1297-319X(02)00450-5.
12. Nienhaus A, Skudlik C, Seidler A (2005) Work-related accidents and occupational diseases in veterinarians and their staff. Int Arch Occup Environ Health 78: 230–238. doi:10.1007/s00420-004-0583-5.
13. Poole AG, Shane SM, Kearney MT, McConnell DA (1999) Survey of occupational hazards in large animal practices. J Am Vet Med Assoc 215: 1433–1435.
14. Landercasper J, Cogbill TH, Strutt PJ, Landercasper BO (1988) Trauma and the veterinarian. J Trauma 28: 1255–1259.
15. Jeyaretnam J, Jones H (2000) Physical, chemical and biological hazards in veterinary practice. Aust Vet J 78: 751–758.
16. Norwood S, McAuley C, Vallina VL, Fernandez LG, McLarty JW, et al. (2000) Mechanisms and patterns of injuries related to large animals. J Trauma 48: 740–744.
17. Deutsches Tierärzteblatt (2012) Statistik 2011: Tierärzteschaft in der Bundesrepublik Deutschland. Available: http://www.freie-berufe-berlin.de/vfb.de/Verweisseiten-VFB/Tieraerzte_2011. Accessed 23 June 2013.
18. Kuorinka I, Jonsson B, Kilbom A, Vinterberg H, Biering-Sørensen F, et al. (1987) Standardised Nordic questionnaires for the analysis of musculoskeletal symptoms. Appl Ergon 18: 233–237. doi:10.1016/0003-6870(87)90010-X.
19. Kristensen TS, Hannerz H, Høgh A, Borg V (2005) The Copenhagen Psychosocial Questionnaire–a tool for the assessment and improvement of the psychosocial work environment. Scand J Work Environ Health 31: 438–449.
20. Kristensen TS, Borritz M, Villadsen E, Christensen KB (2005) The Copenhagen Burnout Inventory: A new tool for the assessment of burnout. Work Stress 19: 192–207. doi:10.1080/02678370500297720.
21. Nübling M, Stößel U, Hasselhorn H-M, Michaelis M, Hofmann F (2006) Measuring psychological stress and strain at work - Evaluation of the COPSOQ Questionnaire in Germany. GMS Psycho-Soc Med 3. Available:/pmc/articles/PMC2736502/?report = abstract. Accessed 20 May 2013.
22. Stoltzfus JC (2011) Logistic Regression: A Brief Primer. Acad Emerg Med 18: 1099–1104. doi:10.1111/j.1553-2712.2011.01185.x.
23. Meers C, Dewulf J, De Kruif A (2008) Work-related accidents and occupational diseases in veterinary practice in Flanders (Belgium). Vlaams Diergeneeskd Tijdschr 77: 40.
24. Lipscomb J, Trinkoff A, Brady B, Geiger-Brown J (2004) Health Care System Changes and Reported Musculoskeletal Disorders Among Registered Nurses. Am J Public Health 94: 1431–1435. doi:10.2105/AJPH.94.8.1431.
25. Walker-Bone K, Palmer KT (2002) Musculoskeletal disorders in farmers and farm workers. Occup Med 52: 441–450.
26. Oude Hengel KM, Visser B, Sluiter JK (2011) The prevalence and incidence of musculoskeletal symptoms among hospital physicians: a systematic review. Int Arch Occup Environ Health 84: 115–119. doi:10.1007/s00420-010-0565-8.
27. Losa Iglesias ME, Becerro De Bengoa Vallejo R, Salvadores Fuentes P (2011) Self-reported musculoskeletal disorders in podiatrists at work. Med Lav 102: 502–510.
28. Beermann B, Brenscheidt F, Siefer A (2007) Arbeitsbedingungen in Deutschland - Belastungen, Anforderungen und Gesundheit. Available: http://www.baua.de/cae/servlet/contentblob/672584/publicationFile/48431/GIZ2005-Arbeitsbedingungen.pdf. Accessed 20 May 2013.
29. Roquelaure Y, Ha C, Leclerc A, Touranchet A, Sauteron M, et al. (2006) Epidemiologic surveillance of upper-extremity musculoskeletal disorders in the working population. Arthritis Care Res 55: 765–778.
30. Gabel CL, Gerberich SG (2002) Risk factors for injury among veterinarians. Epidemiol Camb Mass 13: 80–86.
31. Wijnhoven HAH, de Vet HCW, Picavet HSJ (2006) Prevalence of musculoskeletal disorders is systematically higher in women than in men. Clin J Pain 22: 717–724. doi:10.1097/01.ajp.0000210912.95664.53.
32. De Zwart BCH, Broersen JPJ, Frings-Dresen MHW, Kilbom Å (2000) Gender differences in upper extremity musculoskeletal complaints in the working population. Int Arch Occup Environ Health 74: 21–30. doi:10.1007/s004200000188.
33. Toomingas A, Németh G, Alfredsson L (1995) Self-administered examination versus conventional medical examination of the musculoskeletal system in the neck, shoulders, and upper limbs. J Clin Epidemiol 48: 1473–1483.
34. Lee CE, Simmonds MJ, Novy DM, Jones S (2001) Self-reports and clinician-measured physical function among patients with low back pain: a comparison. Arch Phys Med Rehabil 82: 227–231. doi:10.1053/apmr.2001.18214.
35. Michel A, Kohlmann T, Raspe H (1997) The association between clinical findings on physical examination and self-reported severity in back pain. Results of a population-based study. Spine 22: 296–303.
36. Langley RL, Hunter JL (2001) Occupational fatalities due to animal-related events. Wilderness Environ Med 12: 168–174.
37. Epp T, Waldner C (2012) Occupational health hazards in veterinary medicine: physical, psychological, and chemical hazards. Can Vet J Rev Vétérinaire Can 53: 151–157.
38. Randall E, Hansen C, Gilkey D, Patil A, Bachand A, et al. (2012) Evaluation of ergonomic risk factors among veterinary ultrasonographers. Vet Radiol Ultrasound 53: 459–464. doi:10.1111/j.1740-8261.2012.01942.x.
39. De Zwart BC, Frings-Dresen MH, van Dijk FJ (1995) Physical workload and the aging worker: a review of the literature. Int Arch Occup Environ Health 68: 1–12.
40. Kostelnik K, Heuwieser W (2009) Changing faces of veterinary medicine - shortage of food animal veterinarians. Dtsch Tierärztliche Wochenschr 116: 412–420.
41. Scuffham A, Firth E, Stevenson M, Legg S (2010) Tasks considered by veterinarians to cause them musculoskeletal discomfort, and suggested solutions. N Z Vet J 58: 37–44. doi:10.1080/00480169.2010.64872.
42. DeForge DH (2002) Physical ergonomics in veterinary dentistry. J Vet Dent 19: 196–200.
43. Hayes M, Cockrell D, Smith DR (2009) A systematic review of musculoskeletal disorders among dental professionals. Int J Dent Hyg 7: 159–165. doi:10.1111/j.1601-5037.2009.00395.x.
44. Bongers PM, Ijmker S, van den Heuvel S, Blatter BM (2006) Epidemiology of work related neck and upper limb problems: psychosocial and personal risk factors (part I) and effective interventions from a bio behavioural perspective (part II). J Occup Rehabil 16: 279–302. doi:10.1007/s10926-006-9044-1.
45. Kristensen TS, Bjorner JB, Christensen KB, Borg V (2004) The distinction between work pace and working hours in the measurement of quantitative demands at work. Work Stress 18: 305–322. doi:10.1080/02678370412331314005.
46. Harling M, Strehmel P, Schablon A, Nienhaus A (2009) Psychosocial stress, demoralization and the consumption of tobacco, alcohol and medical drugs by veterinarians. J Occup Med Toxicol Lond Engl 4: 4. doi:10.1186/1745-6673-4-4.

Wirth *et al. Journal of Occupational Medicine and Toxicology* (2016) 11:26
DOI 10.1186/s12995-016-0116-7

Journal of Occupational
Medicine and Toxicology

RESEARCH

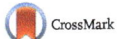

Health behaviour, health status and occupational prospects of apprentice nurses and kindergarten teachers in Germany: a cross-sectional study

Tanja Wirth[1*], Agnessa Kozak[2], Grita Schedlbauer[1] and Albert Nienhaus[1,2]

Abstract

Background: Apprentices in human service professions are exposed to emotional and physical stresses in their workplaces. Moreover, they are in the vulnerable phase of becoming an adult. Their lifestyle and health therefore seem to be particularly unstable. This study aims to evaluate and compare the health behaviour, health status and occupational prospects of apprentices in nursing and early childhood education and to identify factors associated with their physical and mental health.

Methods: A cross-sectional study based on self-administered questionnaires was carried out at eight vocational schools in Hamburg, Germany. Four hundred two apprentice geriatric nurses, hospital nurses and kindergarten teachers/assistants participated (response rate: 99 %). Apprentices were compared in terms of their physical activity, dietary patterns, cigarette and alcohol consumption, body mass index, self-rated health, previous diseases, job satisfaction and occupational prospects. Factors associated with the participants' musculoskeletal or mental disorders were identified using logistic regression.

Results: Around 33 % of apprentice geriatric nurses and kindergarten teachers/assistants were overweight or obese. Fifty-five percent of geriatric nurses were smokers. Job satisfaction was lowest among hospital nurses. More than one third of the apprentices suffered from musculoskeletal or mental disorders. The ages of 23–26 years and mental disorder were associated with musculoskeletal disorders (OR 3.1, 95 % CI 1.4–6.7; OR 1.8, 95 % CI 1.1–3.1). Being an apprentice in early childhood education was associated with an increased chance of mental disorder (OR 2.9, 95 % CI 1.4–6.0). Additionally, musculoskeletal disorders, self-efficacy and irritation were associated with mental disorder.

Conclusions: Differences between the occupational groups indicate the need for specific work-related health promotion for apprentices at an early stage in their careers. Future projects should focus on the implementation and evaluation of these measures.

Keywords: Health behaviour, Health status, Job satisfaction, Mental disorder, Musculoskeletal disorders, Observational study, Student nurses

* Correspondence: t.wirth@cvcare.de
[1]Institution for Statutory Accident Insurance and Prevention in the Health and Welfare Services, Department for the Principle of Prevention and Rehabilitation, Pappelallee 33/35/37, 22089 Hamburg, Germany
Full list of author information is available at the end of the article

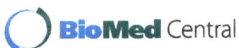

Publikation 2

Wirth *et al. Journal of Occupational Medicine and Toxicology* (2016) 11:26

Page 2 of 10

Background

Hospital and geriatric nurses as well as kindergarten teachers belong to the human service professions, which are becoming increasingly important in our society. Due to an ageing population in the course of demographic change, there is a growing demand for professional nursing care, which will be difficult to cover. Projections estimate that there will be a lack of up to half a million full-time employees in outpatient and inpatient care in Germany by the year 2030 [1]. Similarly, early childhood education has been expanded in Germany in recent years, also leading to a need for more employees in this occupational field. However, nursing professions in particular are not very attractive to graduates. One reason is that these professions are associated with high emotional and physical stress [2]. Besides increasing time pressure at work, dealing with suffering and dying patients is a major challenge in nursing. Kindergarten teachers are exposed to a continuously high level of noise and usually work in bent and twisted postures. Consequently, these professions show high rates of occupational disabilities and dropouts [3, 4], also among young employees [2]. Promoting health early in their careers could be one strategy to prevent high turnover in these professions.

Germany has a practically oriented apprenticeship system. In addition to school education, apprentices spend a large part of their vocational training in the workplace. Thus, apprentices in human service professions are exposed to both performance stress at school and a high degree of stress in their occupations. Moreover, most apprentices are still in the process of becoming an adult, a vulnerable phase in human life, during which one is susceptible to adjusting to an unhealthy lifestyle [5].

Results from the German Health Interview and Examination Survey (DEGS1) indicate that smoking and at-risk drinking are common among a representative sample of young adults aged 18 to 29 years. Forty percent of women in this youngest age group smoked; 36 % consumed alcohol at hazardous levels [6, 7]. According to the DEGS1, 30 % of young women in Germany are overweight [8].

Studies of students in general nursing support the concerns that they also do not follow a healthy lifestyle. A systematic review showed that the smoking rates among nursing students vary considerably depending on the country of study; from 3 % in Iran, to around 30 % in Great Britain, to over 60 % reported in one Australian survey [9]. With regard to Germany, studies consistently reported high smoking rates of over 40 % [10–15]. In a Scottish survey, 74 % of student nurses and midwives practiced harmful alcohol consumption [16]. Around one third of nursing students in Germany consumed alcohol at harmful levels [10]. The highest proportion (45 %) of overweight and obesity among nursing students was found in the US [17]. Rates reported by German studies of

apprentices in the nursing field ranged from 20 to 32 % [12, 13]. A German survey reported that 58 % of apprentices at nursing schools consumed fast food at least once a week [14]. Symptoms of musculoskeletal disorders (MSD) and mental disorders such as depression or burnout have also been observed among nursing students [18, 19].

In Germany, separate vocational training is offered for the two disciplines of geriatric and hospital nursing. Most studies do not distinguish between these two professions; to the best of our knowledge, differentiated analyses among students with respect to health behaviour and health status are missing. Studies examining the health status and behaviour of young apprentices in early childhood education are also lacking. However, analyses of older employees in childcare showed that kindergarten teachers were less likely to be smokers compared to the general German population. In the same study, the prevalence rates for overweight and obesity were 41 and 18 % respectively [20]. Similarly, a study from Georgia reported that 50 % of female childcare providers were overweight or obese [21]. Most early childhood workers in a study from New Zealand believed that they have good nutrition and perceived their health as good or excellent. However, they reported an increase in physical symptoms, such as back pain, muscle strain and fatigue, since they started working in this setting [3].

Dual vocational training at schools and in workplaces provides a unique opportunity for the implementation of health promotion programmes that may increase the awareness of a healthy lifestyle and reduce the effects of occupational stresses. To identify needs for specific measures at vocational schools and workplaces, the health behaviour and status of apprentices must be determined. We have chosen the professions of geriatric nurses, hospital nurses and kindergarten teachers/assistants, as they work in settings with high emotional and physical demands; the constant and intense interactions with patients/clients require a high level of dedication and empathy. In addition, apprentices in these professions serve as role models for patients/clients with respect to their health behaviour. All three occupations also have in common the fact that they are mostly practiced by women and share the same required level of education (general certificate of secondary education).

The objectives of this study were (i) to describe the health status, health behaviour and prospects of apprentice geriatric nurses, hospital nurses and kindergarten teachers/assistants, (ii) to examine differences between these three groups and (iii) to identify factors associated with MSD and mental disorders of apprentices.

Methods

Study design, participants and procedures

A cross-sectional survey was carried out in Hamburg, Germany. Apprentice geriatric nurses, hospital nurses

Wirth *et al. Journal of Occupational Medicine and Toxicology* (2016) 11:26

and kindergarten teachers/assistants were eligible for inclusion in the study. Apprentices in all years of vocational training, of both sexes and all ages were included at this stage. We calculated an estimate of the required sample size based on the prevalence of overweight, as defined by the body mass index (BMI). Overweight is an indicator for health behaviour and a factor influencing the health status. A mean prevalence of 30 % of overweight was assumed among apprentices [12, 13]. For a 95 % chance of our sample estimate being within five percentage points of this assumed prevalence (30 ± 5 %), a sample size of $n = 322$ was needed. We oversampled by 20 % in order to account for non-response and missing data. We therefore aimed to recruit approximately 403 apprentices.

Sixteen out of 20 vocational schools in Hamburg identified for the target professions were contacted at random. Eight of them gave their consent to participate in the study. The schools were responsible for selecting classes by convenience in which questionnaires could be distributed to apprentices during lessons. Apprentices were informed by a project member of the aim and content of the study, of measures to ensure confidentiality and of the voluntary nature of participation. By completing the questionnaires, participants provided their informed consent to take part in the study. Ethical approval was obtained from the Hamburg Medical Council Ethics Committee (# PV4649).

Data collection took place from January to March 2014. In total, 402 apprentices participated in the study (response rate: 98.8 %). The recruitment process is shown in Fig. 1. The age of participants varied greatly from 16 to

52 years. The health behaviour of younger apprentices differs considerably from that of older ones. For example, apprentices under the age of 30 years showed hazardous alcohol consumption ($\chi^2 = 9.9$ [df = 1], p <0.01) and unfavourable dietary patterns ($\chi^2 = 11.4$ [df = 2], p <0.01) significantly more often than their older counterparts. The study sample was therefore reduced to participants aged 16 to 30 years ($n = 354$). We set the cut-off at the age of 30 years to ascertain its comparability with the age group of 18 to 29-year-olds applied in the DEGS1 survey [6–8].

Measures

A self-administered questionnaire was compiled from validated scales and single items which were applied in previous studies. An overview of the scales and items used in the analyses is given in Table 1. The internal consistencies of the self-efficacy, irritation and job satisfaction scale were good (Cronbach's α = 0.81 to 0.88) and comparable to validation studies [22–24]. The applicability and comprehensibility of the instrument was verified in a pre-test with one class of apprentice geriatric nurses ($n = 15$). This class was not included in the final study sample.

Information on the socio-demographic characteristics of participants included age, sex, height, weight, migration background, socioeconomic status (SES) and year of education. Apprentices were classified according to their BMI (kg/m^2) as underweight (<18.5), normal weight (18.5 to 24.9), overweight (25 to 30) or obese (≥30). Migration background was assumed if apprentices themselves had immigrated to Germany and at least one of their parents was not born in Germany or was not of German nationality, or if both parents had immigrated or were not of German nationality [25]. The SES was determined from the highest educational level of apprentices and the current parental occupation. The following scores were administered to educational levels: 1 = comprehensive school qualification, 2 = general certificate of secondary education, 3 = technical college entrance qualification, 4 = university entrance qualification and 5 = technical college entrance qualification or university entrance qualification plus university degree. Parents' occupations were coded according to the International Standard Classification of Occupations (ISCO-88) [26]. By using the International Socio-Economic Index of Occupational Status (ISEI), values from 16 to 90 were assigned to these codes [27]. Scoring categories were defined by quintiles. Scores for educational level were added to scores for the parental occupation with the higher ISEI value. The SES was classified as low (2 to 4), middle (5 to 7) or high (8 to 10) [28].

The health behaviour of apprentices was assessed by physical activity, dietary patterns, smoking habits and

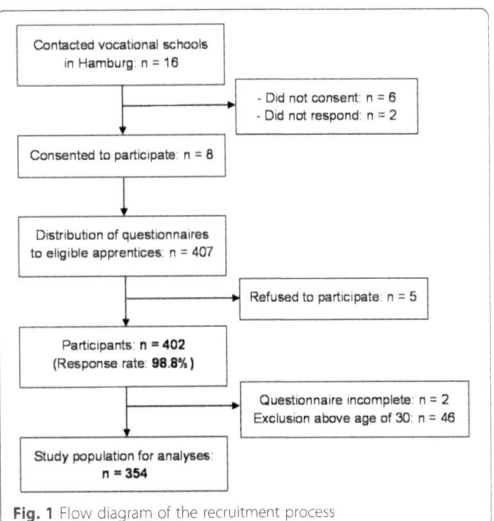

Fig. 1 Flow diagram of the recruitment process

Wirth *et al. Journal of Occupational Medicine and Toxicology* (2016) 11:26

Table 1 Variables of the study instrument used in the analyses

Variables	Name and source of the original scales and items	α	Items (n)
Socio-demographic factors[a]			18
Health behaviour			
Physical activity	Health Questionnaire age 18–64 years [29]	–	1
Dietary habits	Food Frequency Questionnaire [30]	–	15
Smoking	Health Questionnaire age 18–64 years [7]	–	2
Alcohol consumption	AUDIT-C [31, 32]	–	3
Health status			
General health status	Survey in vocational schools in Bielefeld [36]	–	1
Diseases and complaints	Work Ability Index – Questionnaire [33]	–	6
Self-efficacy	Self-efficacy scale [24]	0.85	10
Irritation	Irritation scale [22]	0.88	8
Occupational situation and prospects			
Job satisfaction	COPSOQ: German standard version [23, 34]	0.81	7
Job strain and prospects	Additional questions (e.g., taking into account the current work situation, do you want to stay in this profession for the next five years?)	–	3

[a]Included age, sex, height, weight, migration background, socioeconomic status and year of education
α = Cronbach's alpha, *AUDIT-C* Alcohol Use Disorder Identification Test, *COPSOQ* Copenhagen Psychosocial Questionnaire

alcohol consumption. Regular physical activity was defined as a planned, structured and ongoing activity for increasing physical fitness. For the analysis, activity levels were classified as "no physical activity", "up to 2 h/week" and "regularly, at least 2 h/week" [29]. A food frequency scale, ranging from never to daily, was applied to examine the consumption of fifteen food items. Each item had an individual scoring system from 0 = deviant to 2 = optimal. Scores were added together and classified according to the tertiles of the index [30]. A distinction was made between daily, occasional, former and never smokers. Apprentices smoking ≥20 cigarettes/day were classified as heavy smokers [7]. The Alcohol Use Disorder Identification Test (AUDIT-C) was performed to detect hazardous drinking behaviour. The cut-offs were >3 for women and >4 for men [31, 32].

The health status was rated on a five-point scale ranging from "excellent" to "poor". Questions regarding diseases they had experienced during the previous twelve months were adapted from the Work Ability Index. Response categories were predefined as "no", "yes, own opinion" or "yes, physician's diagnosis" [33]. Two scales evaluated mental health. The General Self-Efficacy Scale identifies resources for coping with life's challenges. It consists of ten items on a four-point Likert scale, with higher scores indicating better self-efficacy [24]. The Irritation scale measures emotional and cognitive psychological strain in occupational contexts. A higher score on a seven-point Likert scale reflects greater irritation [22].

Job satisfaction, motivation to stay in the profession, as well as occupational stresses and wishes were considered

as prospects. Job satisfaction was measured by seven items on a four-point Likert scale. Response categories were transformed to 0 = very dissatisfied, 33 = dissatisfied, 66 = satisfied and 100 = very satisfied [23, 34]. Intentions to stay in the profession for the next five years were predefined as "yes", "no" or "don't know". Two open questions asked about occupational stresses and wishes for the work situation. Out of the free texts, entries categories were formed, which were analysed quantitatively.

Statistical analyses

Frequency distributions and percentages as well as means with corresponding standard deviations (SD) were calculated. Differences between the three professional groups were analysed using the chi-square test for categorical variables. Fisher's exact test was performed if the expected cell frequencies were less than five. Mean differences were evaluated using one-way ANOVA and Scheffé post-hoc tests. If assumptions of normal distribution and homogeneity of variance were not met, non-parametric tests were used. Associations between health-related factors and binary outcome variables (MSD and mental disorder) were examined by logistic regression. Firstly, all variables with a significance value of $p < 0.05$ from univariate analyses were included in a hierarchical model. Secondly, variables with p-value <0.25 were added [35]. If the model did not improve significantly through the second step, a final model with all the variables from the first step was calculated using the "enter" method. Odds ratios with corresponding 95 % confidence intervals and explained variances (Nagelkerke's Pseudo R^2) were calculated from logistic regression analyses. Statistical significance was

Wirth *et al. Journal of Occupational Medicine and Toxicology* (2016) 11:26

set at p <0.05. All statistical analyses were performed using SPSS version 20.

Results

The socio-demographic characteristics of the study participants are presented in Table 2. More than 75 % of apprentices were female. Geriatric nurses were slightly older (23.2 SD 3.3 years) than hospital nurses (21.9 SD 2.4 years) and kindergarten teachers/assistants (21.7 SD 3.5 years, p <0.01). Twenty-seven percent of apprentices were overweight or obese. Among geriatric nurses and kindergarten teachers/assistants, this applied to nearly one third. The SES differed significantly between the groups (p <0.001).

More hospital nurses regularly took part in physical activities (37 %, ≥2 h/week) compared to kindergarten teachers/assistants (31 %) and geriatric nurses (25 %, p = 0.16). The dietary patterns of geriatric nurses and kindergarten teachers/assistants tended to be unfavourable

(41 and 46 %) more often than those of hospital nurses (28 %, p <0.05). The proportion of daily and occasional smokers was highest among geriatric nurses (55 %, p <0.01). Twenty-one percent were classified as heavy smokers (≥20 cigarettes per day), whereas only 12 % of hospital nurses and 4 % of kindergarten teachers/assistants were classified as such. Hazardous drinking behaviour was equally common (p = 0.69) (Table 3).

Around half of the apprentices in each occupational group rated their health as good. Between 31 and 49 % of apprentices reported a mental disorder (p <0.05), either in their own opinion or according to a physician's diagnosis. MSD were the second most prevalent complaint, with proportions exceeding 30 % (Table 3). The body regions most frequently affected were the back, knees or knee joints. Kindergarten teachers/assistants had the lowest self-efficacy and highest irritation. Differences between the groups did not reach statistical significance (Table 3). Irritation was significantly higher among apprentices in their third (24.0 SD

Table 2 Characteristics of the study population

Items	Geriatric nursing (n = 130) n (%)	General healthcare and nursing (n = 142) n (%)	Early childhood education (n = 82) n (%)	p-value
Age groups (years)				<0.001
16–19	20 (15.4)	24 (16.9)	24 (29.3)	
20–22	38 (29.2)	62 (43.7)	29 (35.4)	
23–26	46 (35.4)	49 (34.5)	20 (24.4)	
27–30	26 (20.0)	7 (4.9)	9 (11.0)	
Sex				0.07
Female	98 (75.4)	122 (85.9)	63 (76.8)	
Male	32 (24.6)	20 (14.1)	19 (23.2)	
Body mass index				0.15
< 18.5	4 (3.1)	9 (6.3)	7 (8.5)	
18.5–24.9	78 (60.0)	95 (66.9)	45 (54.9)	
25–30	26 (20.0)	26 (18.3)	18 (22.0)	
≥ 30	14 (10.8)	5 (3.5)	6 (7.3)	
Migration background				0.13
No	90 (69.2)	110 (77.5)	57 (69.5)	
Yes	38 (29.2)	28 (19.7)	25 (30.5)	
Socioeconomic status[a]				<0.001
Low	64 (49.2)	25 (17.6)	37 (45.1)	
Middle	52 (40.0)	79 (55.6)	36 (43.9)	
High	4 (3.1)	30 (21.1)	3 (3.7)	
Year of education				<0.001
1st	32 (24.6)	59 (41.5)	29 (35.4)	
2nd	66 (50.8)	35 (24.6)	53 (64.6)	
3rd	32 (24.6)	48 (33.8)	/	

[a]Derived from educational level of apprentices and parental occupation
Missing values: Body mass index n = 21 (5.9 %); Migration background n = 6 (1.7 %); Socioeconomic status n = 24 (6.8 %)

Publikation 2

Wirth *et al. Journal of Occupational Medicine and Toxicology* (2016) 11:26

Page 6 of 10

Table 3 Group comparisons of health behaviour, health status and occupational prospects

Items	Geriatric nursing (n = 130)	General healthcare and nursing (n = 142)	Early childhood education (n = 82)	Chi^2 (df)	p-value
	n (%)	n (%)	n (%)		
Health behaviour					
Physical activity				6.5 (4)	0.16
No physical activity	33 (25.4)	22 (15.5)	18 (22.0)		
< 2 h/week	62 (47.7)	66 (46.5)	39 (47.6)		
≥ 2 h/week	32 (24.6)	52 (36.6)	25 (30.5)		
Dietary patterns				9.9 (4)	<0.05
Unfavourable	53 (40.8)	39 (27.5)	38 (46.3)		
Normal	36 (27.7)	49 (34.5)	22 (26.8)		
Favourable	26 (20.0)	42 (29.6)	18 (22.0)		
Smoking habits				17.6 (6)	<0.01
Daily	58 (44.6)	43 (30.3)	29 (35.4)		
Occasionally	14 (10.8)	7 (4.9)	7 (8.5)		
Former	17 (13.1)	15 (10.6)	5 (6.1)		
Never	41 (31.5)	77 (54.2)	41 (50.0)		
Hazardous alcohol consumption				0.7 (2)	0.69
Yes	53 (40.8)	60 (42.3)	38 (46.3)		
No	72 (55.4)	80 (56.3)	41 (50.0)		
Health status					
Self-rated health status				9.2 (4)	0.06
Excellent/very good	52 (40.0)	55 (38.7)	25 (30.5)		
Good	65 (50.0)	74 (52.1)	40 (48.8)		
Not so good/poor	11 (8.5)	13 (9.2)	17 (20.7)		
Diseases and complaints					
Mental disorder	50 (38.5)	44 (31.0)	40 (48.8)	7.9 (2)	<0.05
MSD	45 (34.6)	52 (36.6)	26 (31.7)	0.5 (2)	0.79
Neurological or sensory disease	47 (36.2)	39 (27.5)	25 (30.5)	2.3 (2)	0.32
Respiratory disease	34 (26.2)	48 (33.8)	23 (28.0)	1.9 (2)	0.38
Skin disease	33 (25.4)	47 (33.1)	23 (28.0)	2.0 (2)	0.37
Injury due to an accident	37 (28.5)	28 (19.7)	25 (30.5)	4.0 (2)	0.13
	Mean (SD)	Mean (SD)	Mean (SD)	F (df1/df2)	p-value
Self-efficacy (10–40)	29.3 (4.5)	29.2 (4.2)	28.1 (4.9)	1.9 (2/338)	0.15
Irritation (8–56)	23.4 (11.1)	21.9 (9.9)	24.7 (10.2)	1.8 (2/343)	0.17
Occupational prospects					
Job satisfaction (0–100)	62.1 (15.9)	57.4 (15.2)	68.2 (16.7)	12.3 (2/350)	<0.001

Missing values: Physical activity n = 5 (1.4 %); Dietary patterns = 31 (8.8 %); Hazardous alcohol consumption n = 10 (2.8 %); Self-rated health status n = 2 (0.6 %)
SD standard deviation, *df* degrees of freedom, *MSD* musculoskeletal disorders

11.6) and second years (24.2 SD 10.5) of education than for those in their first year (21.1 SD 9.4, p <0.05).

Kindergarten teachers/assistants were significantly more satisfied with their job than geriatric and hospital nurses (p <0.001) (Table 3). Moreover, job satisfaction was highest among apprentices in the first year (68.6 SD 13.8), compared to the second (60.6 SD 15.6) and third years of education (53.1 SD 16.9, p <0.001). With respect to occupational stresses, geriatric nurses most frequently reported time pressure and stress (39 %), physical and mental exertion (30 %) as well as a lack of staff (26 %). Besides these aspects, a high proportion of hospital nurses perceived the team situation and interaction with colleagues as burdensome (26 %). Kindergarten teachers/assistants listed

Publikation 2

Wirth *et al. Journal of Occupational Medicine and Toxicology* (2016) 11:26   Page 7 of 10

physical and mental exertion (35 %) as well as working hours (26 %) most often. The majority of them intended to stay in their profession for the next five years (62 %). This also applied to nearly half of geriatric nurses, but only to 36 % of hospital nurses. Motivation to stay in the profession was significantly lower in the third year of education (35 %) than in the second (47 %) and first years (57 %, $p < 0.001$). More than half of apprentices in all occupational groups demanded higher wages and better public standing for their profession. There was a strong wish for more staff among geriatric and hospital nurses (44 and 53 %). Kindergarten teachers/assistants requested an improvement in working atmosphere and teamwork (25 %).

The variables age, SES, mental disorder, irritation and job satisfaction were significantly related to MSD in univariate analyses and therefore included in a logistic regression model. The ages of 23–26 years (OR 3.1, 95 % CI 1.4–6.7) and mental disorder (OR 1.8, 95 % CI 1.1–3.1) were associated with MSD; the model explained 18 % of the variance in the outcome variable (Table 4).

A logistic regression model for the outcome of mental disorder was formed with the variables apprenticeship trade, SES, MSD, self-efficacy, irritation and job satisfaction. Being an apprentice in early childhood education was associated with an increased chance of mental disorder (OR 2.9, 95 % CI 1.4–6.0). Additionally, MSD, self-efficacy and irritation were significantly associated with mental disorder; the model explained 25 % of the variance in the outcome variable (Table 4).

Discussion

This study was the first to provide a comparison of the health of apprentices in nursing professions and early childhood education. Results show that the health behaviour of geriatric nurses and kindergarten teachers/assistants is particularly worrying. Overall, more than one third of participants reported MSD or mental disorder.

In the present study, only 25 % of geriatric nurses were engaged in sports (≥ 2 h/week). This proportion was considerably lower than among young adults aged 18 to 29 years (37 %) in a recent German survey (DEGS1) [29]. We applied a food frequency index to evaluate the dietary patterns of apprentices, which extends beyond a simple enumeration of consumption frequencies. According to this index, around 46 % of kindergarten teachers/assistants had unfavourable dietary patterns, although teaching a healthy diet is part of their curriculum in Germany. The prevalence of overweight and obesity ranged from 22 % for hospital nurses to 31 % for geriatric nurses. These rates were similar to those of the corresponding age group in the general female population in Germany (30 %) [8]. However, apprentices engaged mainly in technical and commercial occupations showed a lower prevalence of overweight and obesity (19 %) [36].

We detected high smoking rates among geriatric nurses (55 %) and kindergarten teachers/assistants (44 %) which exceeded the smoking rate of 40 % found among young female adults in the general population [7]. However, our findings are in line with the results of studies of nursing students in Germany (smoking rates over 40 %) [10–12, 14, 15]. When compared to international studies, our smoking rates were considerably higher [9]. The proportions of apprentices classified as hazardous drinkers ranged from 41 to 46 % in our study. These were slightly higher than in women from the general population aged 18 to 29 years (36 %) [6].

A considerable proportion of apprentices in our study had suffered from MSD during the previous twelve months (32 to 37 %). Also, high prevalence rates (25 to 53 %) were detected by other investigations of nursing students and professionals in early childhood education [3, 14, 18]. We found that apprentices aged 23 to 26 years were more likely to suffer from MSD than younger apprentices (16 to 19 years). However, the ages of 27 to 30 years was not associated with an increased chance of MSD, meaning that we could not prove a consistent age effect. Other investigations confirm an age trend [37, 38]. It cannot be ruled out that our findings result from the narrow categorisation of age groups chosen for the analysis.

In the present analysis, low SES was associated with a low prevalence of MSD. Previous studies have found inconsistent results. A review reported that low SES was associated with a higher prevalence of musculoskeletal pain [39]. One reason for the inconsistencies could be differences in the methods used to measure the SES. Additionally, we observed a significant correlation between age and SES. Therefore, age could have influenced the association between SES and MSD in our study.

An overview of systematic reviews found strong evidence that poor job satisfaction is a risk factor for the development of low back pain in adults aged 18 years and older [40]. In our study, no association between job satisfaction and MSD was found. Job satisfaction has probably not yet had any substantial influence on the physical health of apprentices, as they have just entered the profession.

Mental disorders measured in our study included several symptoms such as depression, anxiety and chronic insomnia. With frequencies between 8 and 18 % of mental disorders confirmed by a physician's diagnosis, we observed higher twelve-month prevalence rates than the survey of the general German population (4 % in adults aged 18 to 29 years). This prevalence included only diagnosed depressions and no other symptoms which could explain the difference in prevalence rates [41]. Nevertheless, our results of mental disorders could indicate that apprentices suffer from high occupational stress in their workplaces and performance stress due to their involvement in exams at vocational schools, since we

Wirth *et al. Journal of Occupational Medicine and Toxicology* (2016) 11:26

Table 4 Variables associated with musculoskeletal and mental disorders

Musculoskeletal disorders (MSD)			
Independent variables	MSD n (%)	Crude OR (95 % CI)	Adjusted OR[a] (95 % CI)
Age (years)			
16–19	17 (25.0)	1	1
20–22	38 (29.7)	1.3 (0.7–2.5)	1.2 (0.6–2.7)
23–26	58 (50.4)	3.1 (1.6–5.9)**	3.1 (1.4–6.7)**
27–30	10 (23.8)	0.9 (0.4–2.3)	1.0 (0.4–2.8)
Socioeconomic status			
High	16 (43.2)	1	1
Middle	67 (40.1)	0.9 (0.4–1.8)	1.0 (0.5–2.2)
Low	31 (24.8)	0.4 (0.2–0.9)*	0.5 (0.2–1.2)
Mental disorder			
No	60 (27.6)	1	1
Yes	62 (46.3)	2.3 (1.4–3.5)***	1.8 (1.1–3.1)*
Irritation (8–56)	/	1.04 (1.02–1.06)**	1.02 (1.00–1.05)
Job satisfaction (0–100)	/	0.98 (0.97–0.99)**	0.99 (0.97–1.01)
Mental disorder			
Independent variables	Mental disorder n (%)	Crude OR (95 % CI)	Adjusted OR[a] (95 % CI)
Apprenticeship trade			
General healthcare and nursing	44 (31.0)	1	1
Geriatric nursing	50 (38.5)	1.4 (0.8–2.3)	1.4 (0.8–2.7)
Early childhood education	40 (50.0)	2.2 (1.3–3.9)**	2.9 (1.4–6.0)**
Socioeconomic status			
High	9 (24.3)	1	1
Middle	73 (43.7)	2.4 (1.1–5.4)*	2.2 (0.9–5.4)
Low	43 (34.7)	1.7 (0.7–3.8)	1.5 (0.6–4.1)
MSD			
No	72 (31.4)	1	1
Yes	62 (50.8)	2.3 (1.4–3.5)***	2.1 (1.2–3.7)**
Self-efficacy (10–40)	/	0.89 (0.85–0.94)***	0.93 (0.87–0.99)*
Irritation (8–56)	/	1.07 (1.05–1.10)***	1.05 (1.02–1.08)**
Job satisfaction (0–100)	/	0.98 (0.97–0.99)**	0.98 (0.97–1.00)

Multivariate logistic regression analysis to determine variables associated with MSD was performed with $n = 318$ participants (Nagelkerke's Pseudo $R^2 = 0.18$).
Multivariate logistic regression analysis to determine variables associated with mental disorder was performed with $n = 310$ participants (Nagelkerke's Pseudo $R^2 = 0.25$)
[a]Adjusted for the other variables in the model
OR odds ratio, *CI* confidence interval; *$p < 0.05$, **$p < 0.01$, ***$p < 0.001$

measured significantly higher irritation among apprentices in the second than in the first year of education. However, we did not control for academic performance in our study.

Kindergarten teachers/assistants had a 2.9-fold chance of experiencing mental disorder compared to hospital nurses. As the apprenticeship of early childhood education is provided by vocational schools without any reimbursement, a high financial burden is placed on apprentices. This could negatively affect their mental health status.

However, differences observed between occupational groups could also be related to the SES. Individuals with a high SES have a lower risk of suffering from mental illnesses [41]. Hospital nurses had a significantly higher SES than the other groups, which could explain their better mental health status. In general, the dependency between SES and apprenticeship trade might have influenced the relationship between SES and mental disorder. In contrast to the literature, no association could be proven for the latter by logistic regression.

Wirth *et al. Journal of Occupational Medicine and Toxicology* (2016) 11:26

MSD and mental disorder were significantly associated in our study, although the direction of causality is unclear. Lewinsohn et al. [42] showed that physical illness was a significant risk factor for depression in older adolescents. There is also strong evidence for the coexistence of physical and mental illnesses in the general population [43].

Strengths and limitations

The use of heterogeneous instruments to measure health behaviour and status makes a comparison of literature difficult, and also limits the generalisability of the results of this study. Because of the cross-sectional design, no conclusions on causal relationships can be drawn. In addition, results are based on self-reports of participants. When validating the food frequency index, Winkler and Döring [30] pointed out that participants tend to overestimate intake of foods with a healthy image. Furthermore, frequencies of overweight in adolescents are underestimated by studies relying on self-report [44]. For that reason, unfavourable dietary patterns as well as overweight and obesity are likely to be even more prevalent than identified by this study. It was not feasible to draw a random sample of apprentices from the participating schools. The decisions of schools on which classes could take part in the study could not be influenced, as these depended on the upcoming practical periods and exams. Since a convenience sampling strategy had to be used, the study sample might not be representative. We calculated ORs to identify factors associated with MSD and mental disorders. However, these ORs should not be interpreted as estimates of relative risks, as the outcomes were frequent and because of the temporal ambiguity due to the cross-sectional design of our study (Table 4).

Limitations due to a non-response bias can be excluded because of the high response rate of 99 %. The number of missing values was under 5 % for nearly all variables. Extensive socio-demographic information on participants was collected in order to identify possible confounders.

Conclusions

According to the results of the study, it seems to be necessary to develop didactically sound teaching units aimed at strengthening the apprentices' health and avoiding risk factors. Among geriatric nurses, a high smoking rate indicates that more information on the consequences of smoking, individual support in stopping smoking and explicit anti-smoking policies at vocational schools are required [9]. Ergonomic working practices should be actively propagated during vocational training to prevent work-related MSD. Adequate financial support during the apprenticeship might help kindergarten teachers/assistants in reducing stress. Good concepts of health promotion at nursing schools in Germany could already be identified through an ideas competition. Examples are an in-house training in kinaesthetics and a regular running training,

accompanied by lessons on anatomy, physiology and nutrition [45]. Such concepts still have to be developed for the field of early childhood education.

Due to the small sample size, the results of this study should be verified. By including a population-based comparison group, it could be possible to distinguish whether apprentices or young adults in general are at higher risk of the investigated disorders. Furthermore, it should be examined whether health status and health behaviour influence the choice of a particular apprenticeship or whether the particular working and learning conditions influence the health status and behaviour of the young adults. In addition to age, apprenticeship trade, self-efficacy and irritation, which were identified as the most important factors associated with MSD or mental disorder, future studies could evaluate muscle activity and endurance, academic performance, major life events and social support for their association with the health status in apprentices [18, 40, 42].

Leaving aside temporal ambiguity, future projects should concentrate on planning and implementing health promotion measures in the three occupational fields, taking into account the particular circumstances of an apprenticeship. Scientific evaluation can ensure the methodological and content-related quality of these measures.

Acknowledgements
The authors would like to thank all the apprentices who participated in the study and the vocational schools for their support. We also thank Prof. Dr. Zita Schillmöller for assistance with statistical analyses and interpretation of data.

Sources of funding
No external funding.

Authors' contributions
TW was responsible for the conception and design of the study, acquisition, analysis and interpretation of data, and was in charge of writing the article. AK participated in the conception and design of the study, analysis and interpretation of data, and the revision of the article for important intellectual content. GS contributed to the conception and design of the study and the revision of the article. AN participated in the conception and design of the study, interpretation of data and the revision of the article. All authors read and approved the final manuscript.

Competing interests
The authors declare that they have no competing interests.

Author details
[1]Institution for Statutory Accident Insurance and Prevention in the Health and Welfare Services, Department for the Principle of Prevention and Rehabilitation, Pappelallee 33/35/37, 22089 Hamburg, Germany. [2]University Medical Centre Hamburg-Eppendorf, Institute for Health Services Research in Dermatology and Nursing, Martinistraße 52, 20246 Hamburg, Germany.

Received: 24 September 2015 Accepted: 11 May 2016
Published online: 21 May 2016

References
1. Rothgang H, Müller R, Unger R. Themenreport "Pflege 2030" - Was ist zu erwarten - Was ist zu tun? Bertelsmann Stiftung. 2012. https://www.bertelsmann-stiftung.de/fileadmin/files/BSt/Publikationen/GrauePublikationen/GP_Themenreport_Pflege_2030.pdf. Accessed 15 Dec 2015.
2. Dathe D, Paul F, Stuth S. Soziale Dienstleistungen: Steigende Arbeitslast trotz Personalzuwachs. WZBrief Arbeit. 2012;12.

Publikation 2

Wirth et al. Journal of Occupational Medicine and Toxicology (2016) 11:26

Page 10 of 10

3. McGrath BJ, Huntington AD. The health and wellbeing of adults working in early childhood education. AJEC. 2007;32:33–8.
4. Simon M, Tackenberg P, Hasselhorn HM, Kümmerling A, Büschner A, Müller BH. Auswertung der ersten Befragung der NEXT-Studie in Deutschland. Bergische Universität Wuppertal; Universität Witten/Herdecke. 2005. http://www.next.uni-wuppertal.de/index.php?artikel-und-berichte-1. Accessed 21 May 2015.
5. Remschmidt H. Adoleszenz - seelische Gesundheit und psychische Krankheit. Dtsch Arztebl Int. 2013;110:423–4.
6. Hapke U, von der Lippe E, Gaertner B. Alcohol consumption, at-risk and heavy episodic drinking with consideration of injuries and alcohol-specific medical advice. Bundesgesundheitsbl. 2013;56:809–13. doi:10.1007/s00103-013-1699-0.
7. Lampert T, von der Lippe E, Müters S. Prevalence of smoking in the adult population of Germany. Bundesgesundheitsbl. 2013;56:802–8. doi:10.1007/s00103-013-1698-1.
8. Mensink GBM, Schienkiewitz A, Haftenberger M, Lampert T, Ziese T, Scheidt-Nave C. Overweight and obesity in Germany. Bundesgesundheitsbl. 2013;56:786–94. doi:10.1007/s00103-012-1656-3.
9. Smith DR. A systematic review of tobacco smoking among nursing students. Nurse Educ Pract. 2007;7:293–302. doi:10.1016/j.nepr.2006.09.003.
10. Hirsch K, Voigt K, Gerlach K, Kugler J, Bergmann A. Tabak-, Alkohol- und Drogenkonsum sowie Impfverhalten von Gesundheits- und KrankenpflegeschülerInnen in Sachsen-Anhalt. HeilberufeSCIENCE. 2010;1:127–32.
11. Kolleck B. Smoking among nursing students. Pflege. 2004;17:98–104. doi:10.1024/1012-5302.17.2.98.
12. Lehmann F, von Lindeman K, Klewer J, Kugler J. BMI, physical inactivity, cigarette and alcohol consumption in female nursing students: a 5-year comparison. BMC Med Educ. 2014;14. doi:10.1186/1472-6920-14-82.
13. von Lindeman K, Kugler J, Klewer J. Ernährungsgewohnheiten, BMI und Diätversuche von Auszubildenden in Gesundheitsfachberufen. HeilberufeSCIENCE. 2011;2:67–70.
14. Schwanke A, Bomball J, Schmitt S, Stöver M, Görres S. Gesundheitsförderung und Prävention in Pflegeschulen - Ergebnisse einer Studie zur bundesweiten Vollerhebung in Pflegeschulen. Pflegewissenschaft. 2011;4:205–12.
15. Neumann P, Klewer J. Health behaviour of trainees in the socially nursing field – A survey at vocational training schools in Saxony. Pflegewissenschaft. 2010;12:672–7.
16. Watson H, Whyte R, Schartau E, Jamieson E. Survey of student nurses and midwives: smoking and alcohol use. Br J Nurs. 2006;15:1212–6. doi:10.12968/bjon.2006.15.22.22557.
17. Singleton EK, Bienemy C, Hutchinson SW, Dellinger A, Rami JS. A pilot study: a descriptive correlational study of factors associated with weight in college nursing students. ABNF J. 2011;22:89–95.
18. Mitchell T, O'Sullivan PB, Burnett A, Straker L, Smith A, Thornton J, et al. Identification of modifiable personal factors that predict new-onset low back pain: a prospective study of female nursing students. Clin J Pain. 2010;26:275–83. doi:10.1097/AJP.0b013e3181cd16e1.
19. Rudman A, Gustavsson JP. Burnout during nursing education predicts lower occupational preparedness and future clinical performance: a longitudinal study. Int J Nurs Stud. 2012;49:988–1001.
20. Hoffmann SW, Tug S, Simon P. Obesity prevalence and unfavorable health risk behaviors among German kindergarten teachers: cross-sectional results of the kindergarten teacher health study. BMC Public Health. 2013;13:927.
21. Baldwin D, Gaines S, Wold JL, Williams A, Leary J. The health of female child care providers: implications for quality of care. J Community Health Nurs. 2007;24:1–17.
22. Mohr G, Müller A, Rigotti T. Normwerte der Skala Irritation: Zwei Dimensionen psychischer Beanspruchung. Diagnostica. 2005;51:12–20.
23. Nübling M, Stößel U, Hasselhorn H, Michaelis M, Hofmann F. Methoden zur Erfassung psychischer Belastungen. Erprobung eines Messinstrumentes (COPSOQ). Bremerhaven: Wirtschaftsverlag NW; 2005.
24. Schwarzer R, Jerusalem M. Skalen zur Erfassung von Lehrer- und Schülermerkmalen. Dokumentation der psychometrischen Verfahren im Rahmen der Wissenschaftlichen Begleitung des Modellversuchs Selbstwirksame Schulen. 1999. http://userpage.fu-berlin.de/~health/self/skalendoku_selbstwirksame_schulen.pdf. Accessed 20 Sept 2015.
25. Lange M, Kamtsiuris P, Lange C, Schaffrath Rosario A, Stolzenberg H, Lampert T. Messung soziodemographischer Merkmale im Kinder- und Jugendgesundheitssurvey (KiGGS) und ihre Bedeutung am Beispiel der Einschätzung des allgemeinen Gesundheitszustands. Bundesgesundheitsbl. 2007;50:578–89.

26. Geis A. Handbuch für die Berufsvercodung. GESIS. 2011. http://www.gesis.org/fileadmin/upload/dienstleistung/tools_standards/handbuch_der_berufscodierung_110304.pdf. Accessed 07 Jan 2016.
27. Ganzeboom H, Treiman D. Internationally comparable measures of occupational status for the 1988 International Standard Classification of Occupations. Soc Sci Res. 1996;25:201–39.
28. Thomas S, Heinrich S, Kühnlein A, Radon K. The association between socioeconomic status and exposure to mobile telecommunication networks in children and adolescents. Bioelectromagnetics. 2010;31:20–7. doi:10.1002/bem.20522.
29. Krug S, Jordan S, Mensink GBM, Müters S, Finger JD, Lampert T. Physical activity: results of the German Health Interview and Examination Survey for Adults (DEGS1). Bundesgesundheitsbl. 2013;56:765–70. doi:10.1007/s00103-012-1661-6.
30. Winkler G, Döring A. Kurzmethoden zur Charakterisierung des Ernährungsmusters: Einsatz und Auswertung eines Food-Frequency-Fragebogens. Ernährungs-Umschau. 1995;42:289–91.
31. Bush K, Kivlahan DR, McDonell MB, Fihn SD, Bradley KA. The AUDIT Alcohol Consumption Questions (AUDIT-C): an effective brief screening test for problem drinking. Arch Intern Med. 1998;158:1789–95.
32. Reinert DF, Allen JP. The alcohol use disorders identification test: an update of research findings. Alcohol Clin Exp Res. 2007;31:185–99. doi:10.1111/j.1530-0277.2006.00295.x.
33. Hasselhorn HM, Freude G. Der Work Ability Index - ein Leitfaden. Bremerhaven: Wirtschaftsverlag NW; 2007.
34. Kristensen TS, Hannerz H, Hogh A, Borg V. The Copenhagen Psychosocial Questionnaire-a tool for the assessment and improvement of the psychosocial work environment. Scand J Work Environ Health. 2005;31:438–49.
35. Hosmer DW, Lemeshow S. Applied logistic regression. New York: John Wiley & Sons; 2000.
36. Kaminski A, Nauerth A, Pfefferle PI. Gesundheitszustand und Gesundheitsverhalten von Auszubildenden im ersten Lehrjahr - Erste Ergebnisse einer Befragung in Bielefelder Berufskollegs. Gesundheitswesen. 2008;70:38–46.
37. Bot SD, van der Waal JM, Terwee CB, van der Windt DA, Schellevis FG, Bouter LM, et al. Incidence and prevalence of complaints of the neck and upper extremity in general practice. Ann Rheum Dis. 2005;64:118–23. doi:10.1136/ard.2003.019349.
38. de Zwart BC, Broersen JP, Frings-Dresen MH, van Dijk FJ. Musculoskeletal complaints in the Netherlands in relation to age, gender and physically demanding work. Int Arch Occup Environ Health. 1997;70:352–60.
39. McBeth J, Jones K. Epidemiology of chronic musculoskeletal pain. Best Pract Res Clin Rheumatol. 2007;21:403–25.
40. Lakke SE, Soer R, Takken T, Reneman MF. Risk and prognostic factors for non-specific musculoskeletal pain: a synthesis of evidence from systematic reviews classified into ICF dimensions. Pain. 2009;147:153–64.
41. Busch M, Maske U, Ryl L, Schlack R, Hapke U. Prevalence of depressive symptoms and diagnosed depression among adults in Germany - Results of the German Health Interview and Examination Survey for Adults (DEGS1). Bundesgesundheitsbl. 2013;56:733–9. doi:10.1007/s00103-013-1688-3.
42. Lewinsohn PM, Rohde P, Seeley JR. Major depressive disorder in older adolescents: prevalence, risk factors, and clinical implications. Clin Psychol Rev. 1998;18:765–94.
43. Hogg-Johnson S, van der Velde G, Carroll LJ, Holm LW, Cassidy JD, Guzman J, et al. The burden and determinants of neck pain in the general population. Results of the Bone and Joint Decade 2000–2010 Task Force on Neck Pain and Its Associated Disorders. Spine. 2008;3:39–51.
44. Sherry B, Jefferds ME, Grummer-Strawn LM. Accuracy of adolescent self-report of height and weight in assessing overweight status: a literature review. Arch Pediatr Adolesc Med. 2007;161:1154–61. doi:10.1001/archpedi.161.12.1154.
45. Görres S, Stöver M, Bomball J, Schwanke A, Bremer M, Adrian C. Bundesweiter Ideenwettbewerb "Gesunde Pflegeausbildung". Anwendungsbeispiele für die Praxis Universität Bremen: IPP Schriften. 2012;10.

Kozak et al. BMC Musculoskeletal Disorders (2015) 16:231
DOI 10.1186/s12891-015-0685-0

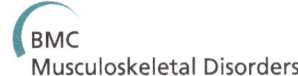

BMC
Musculoskeletal Disorders

RESEARCH ARTICLE

Open Access

CrossMark

Association between work-related biomechanical risk factors and the occurrence of carpal tunnel syndrome: an overview of systematic reviews and a meta-analysis of current research

Agnessa Kozak[1*], Grita Schedlbauer[2†], Tanja Wirth[2†], Ulrike Euler[3], Claudia Westermann[1] and Albert Nienhaus[1,2†]

Abstract

Background: Occupational risks for carpal tunnel syndrome (CTS) have been examined in various occupations, and several systematic reviews (SRs) have been published on this topic. There has been no critical appraisal or synthesis of the evidence in the SRs. The aims of this study are (1) to synthesise the observational evidence and evaluate the methodological quality of SRs that assess the effect of biomechanical risk factors on the development of CTS in workers, (2) to provide an update of current primary research on this association, (3) to assess a potential dose-response relationship.

Methods: We searched MEDLINE, EMBASE, CINAHL, the Cochrane Library and the reference lists of articles. The first step covered SRs (1998–2014), and the second step covered current primary studies (2011–2014). The methodological quality of the SRs was evaluated by using the AMSTAR-R tool; primary studies were assessed using a list of 20 items. A qualitative approach was used for synthesising evidence. In addition, we undertook a meta-analysis of the primary studies to determine risk ratios in the dose-response relationship.

Results: We identified ten SRs that covered a total of 143 original studies. Seven primary studies met the criteria for inclusion, of which four provided longitudinal data. We found high quality of evidence for risk factors such as repetition, force and combined exposures. Moderate quality of evidence was observed for vibration, and low quality of evidence was found for wrist postures. An association between computer use and CTS could not be established. Recent primary studies supported the existence of a significant relationship between CTS and repetition, force and combined exposure. The meta-analysis of current research revealed a dose-response relationship between CTS and the American Conference of Governmental Industrial Hygienists' (ACGIH) threshold limit value (TLV) for hand-activity level (HAL). Those between the action limit and TLV and above TLV had RR of 1.5 (95 % CI 1.02–2.31) and RR 2.0 (95 % CI 1.46–2.82), respectively.

Conclusions: Occupational biomechanical factors play a substantial role in the causation of CTS. Data from current primary studies on dose-response suggest that the risk of CTS increases with the ACGIH TLV levels.

Background

Carpal tunnel syndrome (CTS) is a pathophysiological peripheral mononeuropathy, caused by an increase in the tissue pressure in the carpal tunnel. This leads to pressure damage of the N. medianus, linked to sensory and motor failures in the affected area. CTS is the most frequent compression syndrome of a peripheral nerve. A review of occupational populations showed that the prevalence of CTS varies greatly with the diagnostic criteria, population and study type, and it may range from 0.6 to 61 % [1, 2]. In population-based studies, the prevalence rates range from 1 to 6 % [3–6]. CTS mainly affects women and increases with age. In Swedish and Italian population studies, the annual incidence for women was 428 and 506 per 100,000 respectively. This is about three times greater than the corresponding values for men, namely 182 and 139 cases per 100,000

* Correspondence: a.kozak@uke.de
†Equal contributors
1Institute for Health Services Research in Dermatology and Nursing (CVcare), University Medical Center Hamburg-Eppendorf, Hamburg, Germany
Full list of author information is available at the end of the article

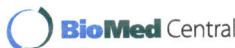

Kozak et al. BMC Musculoskeletal Disorders (2015) 16:231

respectively [7, 8]. The causes of CTS may be local (e.g., cysts), regional (e.g., rheumatoid arthritis) or systemic (e.g., diabetes) [9]. There is increasing scientific evidence that development of CTS is promoted by highly repetitive manual tasks, involving awkward hand/wrist postures, with flexion and extension of the hands, forceful exertion or hand/arm vibration during work [1, 10]. Some occupational groups are more exposed than others, due to the nature of their work. These are mostly occupations requiring the frequent use of hand-held vibratory tools and high levels of physical exposure, particularly during assembly work, food processing and packaging [11]. As CTS is common in the general population and is multi-causal, it is legitimate to ask to what extent it is caused by occupational factors. This has been a controversial issue for many years [12–16]. For example, Thurston [17] argued that occupational factors — such as repetition, vibration or force — are not the primary cause of CTS and that it was more likely that these activities trigger symptoms or exacerbate existing latent symptoms. In a prospective study on the aetiology of CTS in the industrial sector, the authors found out that individual factors, such as age, being overweight, gender, hand anthropometrics and hand dominance play a much greater role in causing CTS than occupational factors, such as force, repetition, duration of employment and type of employment [18–20]. However, early systematic reviews (SRs) concluded that there is sufficient evidence for an association between occupational exposure to biomechanical factors and the development of CTS [1, 10, 21, 22].

In recent years, several SRs and meta-analyses have been published on the aetiology of CTS in the occupational context. There has however been no critical evaluation of the SRs or a discussion of the results. The "overview of systematic reviews" represents a new approach to synthesising evidence from several SRs [23]. Overviews can potentially provide a broad summary of empirical research on a specific issue [24]. The information provided by these overviews is essentially dependent on the validity of the primary studies and the SRs that they include [25]. As SRs may very rapidly become dated, it is advisable to include the most recent publications, too [26, 27].

This overview aims to synthesise and critically evaluate the quality of SRs and current primary studies assessing the relationship between occupational biomechanical factors and CTS in working populations. Another objective is to quantify the dose-response relationship using the American Conference of Governmental Industrial Hygienists (ACGIH) threshold limit value (TLV) for hand-activity level (HAL) model.

Methods

The literature search and analysis took place in two steps. The first step consisted of an explicit search for SRs. The procedure was based on the methods paper published by the Clearinghouse of Systematic Reviews of the Partnership for European Research in Occupational Safety and Health (PEROSH) [28]. In the second step, primary studies were identified and evaluated. This study was conducted according to the Meta-analysis of Observational Studies in Epidemiology (MOOSE) checklist (see Additional file 1) [29].

Search strategy and study selection

An electronic literature search for SRs was performed in the MEDLINE (via Pubmed), EMBASE (via Ovid), CINAHL (via EBSCO) and COCHRANE databases. It covered the publication period from 1998 to 2014 (last update 27.7.14) and used predefined search strings and terms. In order to identify aetiological studies in the occupational context, we employed the sensitive search string developed by Mattioli et al. [30], in combination with the terms for exposure (exposure; physical load; risk factor*; repetiti*; hand-arm vibration; force), outcome (carpal tunnel syndrome; median nerve neuropathy; median nerve entrapment; nerve compression syndrome) and study design (meta-analysis; review; not letter, editorial, comment). The search strategy is listed in the Additional file 2. We also searched for additional sources within the references of relevant publications. The following inclusion and exclusion criteria for SRs were applied:

- Population: employed adults.
- Exposure: biomechanical factors in the occupational context (exclusion: studies on diagnostic testing, treatment or rehabilitation).
- Outcome: CTS as primary outcome (exclusion: CTS as concomitant disease, e.g., in diabetes mellitus).
- Design: SRs and meta-analyses (exclusion: narrative reviews, editorials, commentaries).

To update the analysis, we conducted a primary literature search using MEDLINE, EMBASE and CINAHL databases. The same sensitive search string was employed, except for the partial string for SRs and meta-analyses. The last comprehensive literature search was performed in the meta-analysis published by Spahn et al. [31]. Our search therefore included the period January 2011 to 2014 (last update 31.8.2014). The following inclusion and exclusion criteria were applied for primary studies:

- Population: employed adults.
- Exposure: consideration of at least one biomechanical exposure factor, giving degrees of association or raw data.
- Outcome: conservative CTS case definition: (a) abnormal findings in the nerve conduction study

Publikation 3

Kozak *et al. BMC Musculoskeletal Disorders* (2015) 16:231

Page 3 of 19

(NCS) that indicated dysfunction of the N. medianus in the carpal tunnel and (b) either clinical signs (a positive Phalen's or Tinel's sign) or symptoms indicative of CTS such as paraesthesia, numbness or pain.
- Design: peer review article with case control, cross-sectional and cohort studies.

Six languages (English, German, Italian, Spanish, Portuguese and Russian) were considered. The studies were selected independently by two reviewers (AK, TW). In the event of disagreement, consensus was achieved by discussion. When no consensus could be achieved, a third reviewer (GS) was consulted. Data were extracted by one reviewer (AK). To verify accuracy of extraction, a second and a third reviewer (TW, GS) checked all relevant data for each included SR and primary study. Data extracted from the studies is listed in the Additional file 3.

Degree of overlap between the SRs

If primary studies are included in more than a single SR on the same research question, this can lead to bias in the interpretation of the results of the overview. For this reason, it was necessary for the overview to determine the extent to which the primary studies overlapped in the different SRs. This is presented in Table 1. Additionally, a calculation was performed of the percentage of primary studies included in more than one SR. A measure of overlap was also calculated — the "Corrected Covered Area" (CCA), using the method proposed by Pieper et al. [26]. The included primary studies were extracted from each SR, documented and calculated in an Excel table (SR x primary studies). CCA can be interpreted as the overlap area of studies that occur at least twice in SRs, after correction for the first time each

primary study was counted (index publications). The frequency of repeated occurrence of index publications in SRs (N) is divided by the product of index publications (r) and reviews (c), minus by the number of index publications (r; see calculation formula). CCA values between 0 and 5 indicate slight overlap; values between 6 and 10 moderate overlap, values between 11 and 15 high overlap and values above 15 very high overlap [26].

$$CCA = \frac{N-r}{rc-r}$$

N is the number of publications included (with duplicate counts) in the evidence synthesis of individual SRs; r is the number of index publications (individual primary studies) and c the number of SRs.

Quality assessment

The validity of the included SRs was critically and independently assessed by two reviewers using the Assessment of Multiple Systematic Reviews – Revised (AMSTAR-R), an instrument that was specifically developed to assess the methodological quality of SRs [32]. Between 11 and 44 points could be reached on the AMSTAR-R score. To differentiate between the SRs, the numerical score was converted to quality grades: $A = 37–44$ (very good); $B = 29–36$ (good); $C = 21–28$ (moderate); $D = 13–20$ (poor) points [33]. The inter-rater reliability between two reviewers was determined with Cohen's kappa coefficient [34].

The evaluation of the validity of the primary studies was based on the criteria developed by van Rijn et al. [35] and Ariëns et al. [36] (see Additional file 4). These were adapted to suit the research question and then summarised to a cumulative score with a maximum of 20 points. Quality was rated as methodologically

Table 1 Overlap of original research studies included in the systematic reviews

Author, year	1	2	3	4	5	6	7	8	9	10
1. Abbas et al. 1998 [21]	**17**	0	9	1	7	10	9	8	3	0
2. Sulsky et al. 2005 [44]		**34**	12	3	12	14	6	13	0	3
3. Palmer et al. 2007 [22]			**38**	5	19	18	16	19	4	2
4. Thomsen et al. 2008 [45]				**9**	4	4	1	3	1	3
5. Lozano-Calderón et al. 2008ª [46]					**66**	18	12	16	5	2
6. van Rijn et al. 2009 [35]						**44**	21	21	3	3
7. Barcenilla et al. 2012 [41]							**37**	22	3	0
8. Spahn et al. 2012ª [31]								**55**	2	1
9. You et al. 2014 [43]									**8**	0
10. Mediouni et al. 2014 [42]										**6**

Bold numbers are studies included in each SRs
ªIncluded primary studies that were used for the analysis of occupational risk factors, but which were not listed explicitly, e.g., in the form of an evidence table. Consequently all studies from all tables, figures or text were extracted when they were used for the analysis of occupational factors. This was used to determine overlap

Kozak *et al. BMC Musculoskeletal Disorders* (2015) 16:231

high (≥14 points), moderate (8 to 13 points) or poor (≤7 points).

Quality of evidence

Due to the heterogeneity of the primary studies and the overlap of the study pool of the SRs included, no formal evidence synthesis was possible with the Grades of Recommendation, Assessment, Development and Evaluation (GRADE) approach [37]. We therefore determined the quality of evidence using a qualitative approach for each type of occupational exposure. The assessment of the quality of evidence depended on the methodological validity of the SRs (AMSTAR-R score), together with the consistency of the results between the SRs (direction of effect and significance) [38, 39]. We gave greater weight to recently published SRs; older SRs provided supportive evidence [27]. The following classification was specified:

- High – consistent evidence in very good SRs (at least one grade A review).
- Moderate – consistent evidence in good SRs (at least one grade B review).
- Low – one SR of moderate quality (at least grade C) and significant results and/or good SRs (grade B), with some inconsistent results.
- Poor – none of the above conditions were met (i.e., consistent findings in low-quality SRs (grade D), or inconsistent findings in multiple SRs).

The results of the primary studies served to support the assessment of the quality of evidence, as both their methodological validity and their consistency were considered; i.e., when at least two valid primary studies (≥14 points) gave consistent results, the quality of the evidence from the SRs was upgraded.

Statistical analyses

Comparable primary studies were pooled in the form of quantitative data synthesis and presented as forest plots. The relative risk (RR) was calculated and 95 % confidence intervals (CI) were generated. The heterogeneity of individual studies was quantified using the Chi-square (χ^2) and I^2 statistics. If there was statistically significant heterogeneity (χ^2, $p <0.10$ and $I^2 > 50$ %), then the pooled effect estimate was determined with the random effects model. Otherwise, a fixed effects model was used [40]. The analyses were applied to current primary studies and were conducted using RevMan Version 5.2.

Ethics

Ethical approval was not required as the study focused only on analysing secondary literature without any involvement of human subjects, tissues or medical records.

Results

SRs and meta-analyses

A total of ten relevant SRs were included. The flow diagram (Fig. 1) shows the selection of SRs identified by the electronic and hand search. The number of primary studies per SR varied from 6 to 66. Taken together, the ten SRs covered a total of 143 primary studies (index publications); these were cited up to 314 times in the SRs. 35 % of the index publications were cited in two to three SRs and about 29 % in four to six SRs (Table 1). The CCA value was 13.3, which indicates a high degree of overlap. Table 2 shows the detailed characteristics of the included SRs. In half of the SRs, a meta-analysis was performed [21, 31, 41–43]. Five of the other SRs presented the results qualitatively in the form of an evidence table [22, 35, 44–46]. Two SRs concentrated exclusively on the link between computer use and CTS [42, 45]. A meta-analysis by You et al. [43] only examined the link between non-neutral wrist postures and CTS. The paper by Sulsky et al. [44] is a report from the Occupational Insurance Association for Safety at Work; this was not published as a peer review article.

Using AMSTAR-R scoring, three SRs were categorised as "grade B" [35, 41, 42], five as "grade C" [22, 31, 43–45] and two as "grade D" publications [21, 46]. With a single exception, the inter-rater reliability was good to very good (kappa: 0.38–0.87) (see Additional file 5).

SRs used different instruments and methods to assess the methodological quality of the included studies. The Cochrane Collaboration's tool for assessing risk of bias was used by only a single meta-analysis [41]. Selective criteria were used in three additional studies, which all considered aspects such as study design, allocation of participants, outcome and exposure assessment, as well as the control of potential confounders [35, 44, 45]. You et al. [43] identified possible bias with sensitivity analyses; Mediouni et al. [42] provided the strengths and limitations of the original studies in an evidence table. Lozano-Calderón et al. [46] developed an assessment scheme in accordance with the Bradford-Hill criteria for causality and used this score to determine the quality and the strength of the evidence for the aetiological link between generally accepted risk factors for CTS (biological, occupational, as well as biological and occupational together).

The results from the SRs and meta-analyses are predominantly based on cross-sectional and case control studies; prospective longitudinal studies were in the minority. Table 3 shows the main results from the SRs.

Current primary studies

The selection of the primary studies employed the same selection process as for the SRs. After scrutinising 366 titles and abstracts, we reviewed 49 full texts and

Kozak *et al. BMC Musculoskeletal Disorders* (2015) 16:231

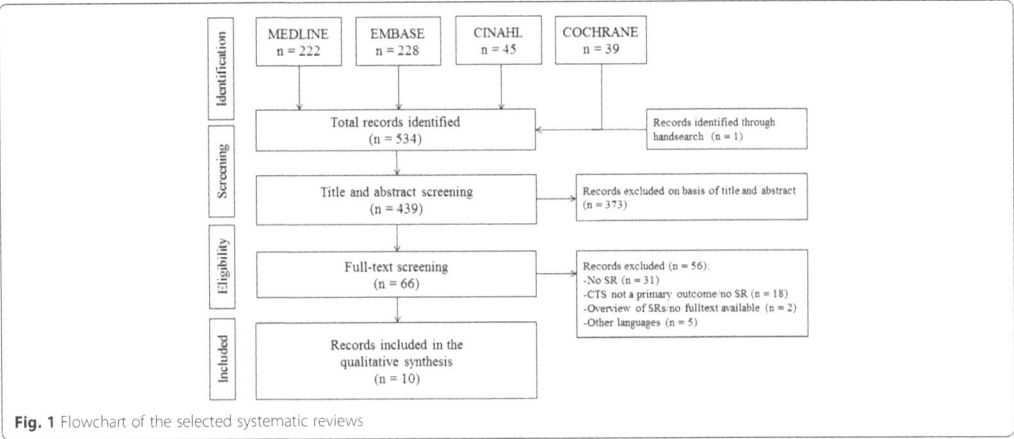

Fig. 1 Flowchart of the selected systematic reviews

included a total of seven studies in the evidence synthesis (Fig. 2). The main reasons for exclusion were no conservative CTS definition (*n* = 20) or no investigation of biomechanical risk factors (*n* = 13). Of the included studies, four were of high quality and had a prospective design [47–50], although one publication only presented the baseline results [48]. The other three studies were of moderate quality, including one prospective study [51] and two case control studies (see Additional file 4) [52, 53]. In four studies, the exposures were measured with objective methods [47–50]. In two studies, exposures were self-reported [52, 53] and in one study, exposures were assessed with Job Exposure Matrices (JEM, US O*NET Database) [51]. A summary of the characteristics of the included primary studies along with the main results are shown in Table 4. All four studies of high quality determined the ACGIH TLV for HAL and were incorporated in the meta-analysis to clarify the dose-response relationship [47–50]. This score includes the combined exposure from peak force (PF) and repetition (HAL). HAL is based on frequency of exertion and duty cycle of exertion. PF is based on the peak effort exerted by the hand during the regular duty cycle. PF and HAL are combined into a single measure by calculating the ratio PF/(10-HAL). As proposed by ACGIH the TLV for HAL score <0.56 is considered below the Action Limit (AL) and is a category for general controls due to low risk. A score >0.78 is considered above the TLV and indicates a high risk. Scores between AL and TLV are considered to be possibly dangerous borderline exposures [54]. For the results of the meta-analysis see the paragraph on combined exposures.

Repetition

Seven SRs (two grade B, three grade C and two grade D) examined repetition as a risk factor for CTS (Table 3).

On the basis of the highest-quality study available, there is a significant association between repetition and CTS. This association is maintained when only studies that used a conservative CTS case definition [41] are considered. A SR of good quality (grade B) showed that five out of eight studies found a positive association with CTS. The authors concluded that cycles times of <10 s were more harmful than cycles times of <30 s, or when the same movements were performed in >50 % of working time [35]. Another meta-analysis also confirmed this association, though this had not been demonstrated for longitudinal studies [31]. A meta-regression analysis by Abbas et al. [21] showed that country, study population, repetition and force were significant predictors of CTS. Sulsky et al. [44] confirmed that there is consistent evidence for a weak positive relationship between CTS and repetition. Palmer et al. [22] also found that there is an increased risk of CTS from highly repetitive flexion and extension of the wrist. Using the Bradford-Hill criteria for causality, Lozano-Calderón et al. [46] found only slight evidence for a causal relationship between repetition and CTS (Bradford-Hill score: 6.5 of 21 points).

All of the included primary studies confirm that there is a positive association between repetition and CTS (Table 4). The baseline results of Burt et al. [48] show an interaction between BMI and the frequency of exertion per minute (≥5 % of the maximal voluntary contraction). High frequency of exertion (≥15 times/min.) resulted in a three-fold higher probability of CTS in the obese (BMI ≥30). Obesity doubled the odds for CTS among those with frequent exertion per minute. Furthermore, a significant association between HAL and CTS was observed for men but not for women (OR 1.4, 95 % CI 1.05–1.81). Bonfiglioli et al. [50] found that HAL was an independent predictor of CTS (IRR 1.4, 95 % CI 1.19–1.57). According to

Publikation 3

Kozak *et al. BMC Musculoskeletal Disorders* (2015) 16:231

Page 6 of 19

Table 2 Study characteristics of the included systematic reviews and meta-analyses

Author, year	Analysis	AMSTAR-R grade	Country	Years included	No. of studies included	Study designs	A priori quality criteria	The study's aim was to …
You et al. 2014 [43]	MA	C	US	1980–2012	n = 8	CC = 2; CS = 6	Recognition of bias by sensitivity analysis	… conduct a meta-analysis of existing studies to evaluate the evidence of the relationship between wrist posture at work and CTS
Mediouni et al. 2014 [42]	MA	B	FR	1992–2012	n = 6	C = 2; CS = 4	Strengths and limitations acknowledged	… conduct a systematic review and meta-analysis of the available epidemiological data on the association between computer work exposure and CTS
Barcenilla et al. 2012 [41]	MA	B	AU	1980–2009	n = 37	C = 3; CC = 5; CS = 28	Risk of Bias Tool	… examine the association between workplace exposure and CTS by meta-analysis, with respect to exposure to hand force, repetition, vibration and wrist posture
Spahn et al. 2012 (in German) [31]	MA	C	DE	≤2011	n = 55	n/a	n/a	… conduct a systematic review and meta-analysis to identify associated and risk factors for CTS in the occupational setting
Van Rijn et al. 2009 [35]	SR	B	NL	1966–2007	n = 44	C = 5; CC = 9; CS = 30	16-item score	… provide a quantitative assessment of the exposure-response relationship between work-related physical and psychosocial factors and the occurrence of CTS in occupational populations
Lozano-Calderón et al. 2008 [46]	SR	D	US	≤2008	n = 51[a], n = 33[b], (total = 66)	C = 7[a]; CC = 12[a], C = 29[a], Other = 3[a]	Bradford Hill criteria for causation	… evaluate the quality and strength of scientific evidence supporting an aetiological relationship between a disease and a proposed risk factor, using a scoring system based on the Bradford Hill criteria for causal association – example of CTS
Thomsen et al. 2008 [45]	SR	C	DK	≤2004	n = 8	C = 4; CC = 2; CS = 2	Selected criteria (4 main domains)	… conduct a systematic review to examine evidence for an association between computer work and CTS
Palmer et al. 2007 [22]	SR	C	GB	≤2004	n = 38	n/a	n/a	… conduct a systematic review to assess occupational risk factors for CTS
Sulsky et al. 2005 [44]	SR	C	DE	1997–2003	n = 34	C = 10; CC = 2; CS = 22	Selected criteria (6 main domains)	… clarify the relationship between CTS and occupation using quality based criteria from the epidemiological literature
Abbas et al. 1998 [21]	MA	D	US	1980–1995	n = 17	C = 3; CC = 4; CS = 10	n/a	… conduct a meta-analysis on work-related CTS and to identify risk estimates and possible biases influencing the risk estimates

Abbreviations: AMSTAR-R Assessment of Multiple Systematic Reviews – Revised (numeric quality score in grades: A = 37–44; B = 29–36; C = 21–28; D = 13–20 points), *C* Cohort, *CC* Case control, *CS* Cross-sectional, *CTS* Carpal tunnel syndrome, *MA* Meta-analysis, *SR* Systematic review
[a]Studies investigating occupational factors alone
[b]Studies investigating both biological and occupational factors

Kozak *et al. BMC Musculoskeletal Disorders* (2015) 16:231

Table 3 Main results of the included systematic reviews and meta-analyses stratified by the exposure factors

Author, year, ↓quality	Vibration (95 % CI)	Repetition (95 % CI)	Force (95 % CI)	Combined exposure (repetition and force) (95 % CI)	Wrist posture (95 % CI)	Computer exposure (95 % CI)
Barcenilla et al. 2012 [41] Grade B	NIOSH CTS def.: OR 2.7 (1.9–3.9); n = 12 studies Conservative CTS def.[a]: OR 5.4 (3.1–9.3); n = 3/3 (100 %) studies[d]	NIOSH CTS def.: OR 2.3 (1.8–3.0); n = 25 studies Conservative CTS def.[a]: OR 2.3 (1.7–2.9); n = 5/11 (45 %) studies[d]	NIOSH CTS def.: OR 2.2 (1.5–3.3); n = 13 studies Conservative CTS def.[a]: OR 4.2 (1.5–11.7); n = 3/5 (60 %) studies[d]	NIOSH CTS def.: OR 2.0 (1.4–2.9); n = 4/9 (44 %) studies[d] Conservative CTS def.[a]: OR 1.9 (1.0–3.5); n = 5 studies	NIOSH CTS def.: OR 2.7 (1.3–5.5); n = 7 studies Conservative CTS def.[a]: OR 4.7 (0.4–53.3); n = 1/3 (33 %) studies[d]	/
Mediouni et al. 2014 [42] Grade B	/	/	/	/	/	Computer use: OR 1.7 (0.8–3.6); n = 5 studies; Keyboard/mouse use: OR 1.1 (0.6–2.0); OR 1.9 (0.9–4.2)
Van Rijn et al. 2009 [35] Grade B	OR 2.5–4.8; n = 3/5 (60 %) studies[d]	OR 0.5–9.4; n = 5/8 (62 %) studies[d]	OR 2.1–9.0; n = 3/7 (43 %) studies[d]	OR 3.2–8.4; n = 3/4 (80 %) studies[d]	OR 1.3–8.7; n = 4/5 (80 %) studies[d]	OR 2.1–4.4; n = 2/7 (29 %) studies[d]
You et al. 2014 [43] Grade C	/	/	/	/	Non-neutral wrist postures: RR 2.0 (1.7–2.4); n = 4/8 (50 %) studies[d]	/
Spahn et al. 2012 [31] Grade C	OR 2.6 (1.7–4.0); n = 6/9 (67 %) studies[d]	OR 2.7 (1.8–3.9); n = 11/13 (85 %) studies[d] OR 2.1 (0.4–11.8); n = 3 cohort studies	OR 4.4 (1.4–13.6); n = 4/4 (100 %) studies[d]	OR 8.4 (7.8–8.9)[b]; n = 2/2 (100 %) studies[d] OR 1.8 (1.4–2.2)[b]; n = 2/3 (67 %) cohort studies[d]	Flexion: OR 1.7 (1.0–2.6); n = 2/5 (40 %) studies[d]	Computer use: OR 1.8 (0.8–4.1); n = n/a studies
Sulsky et al. 2005 [44][c] Grade C	Insufficient evidence; n = 1 study	Consistent small positive association; n = 6 studies	Weak positive association of questionable validity; n = 3 studies	/	Insufficient evidence; n = 1 study	Insufficient evidence; n = 2 studies
Thomsen et al. 2008 [45] Grade C	/	/	/	/	/	Inconsistent evidence: OR < 1; n = 1 studies; OR > 1; n = 3 studies and n = 4 studies with no effect calculation or n.s.
Palmer et al. 2007 [22] Grade C	≥2 OR elevated risk (e.g., exposure ≥8 years); n = 7 studies	≥2 OR elevated risk (e.g., exposure <10 s. cycle time); n = 5 studies	Elevated risk for high-force jobs and activities (e.g., exposure >4 kg); n = n/a studies	Elevated risk for jobs with combined exposure; n = 1 study	≥2 OR elevated risk (e.g., exposure >17 or 20 h/week); n = 4 studies	/
Abbas et al. 1998 [21] Grade D	/	Significant predictor	Significant predictor	/	/	/

Publikation 3

Kozak *et al. BMC Musculoskeletal Disorders* (2015) 16:231

Page 8 of 19

Table 3 Main results of the included systematic reviews and meta-analyses stratified by the exposure factors (*Continued*)

| Lozano-Calderón et al. 2008 [46] Grade D | Ø OR 5.5; qBHs 6.3/21 points (range 5–8); n = 14/20 (70 %) studies[cd] | Ø OR 5.5; qBHs 6.5/21 points (range 5–10); n = 30/45 (67 %) studies[cd] | / | Ø OR n/a; qBHs 4.5/21 points (range 3–6); n = 15/31 (48 %) studies[cd] | Flexion: Ø OR n/a; qBHs 5.4/21 points (range 4–8); n = 7/17 (41 %) studies[cd]
Extension: Ø OR n/a; qBHs 3.6/21 points (range 3–4); n = 3/7 (43 %) studies[cd] | / |

Abbreviations: CI Confidence interval, *CTS* Carpal tunnel syndrome, *NIOSH* National Institute for Occupational Health and Safety (USA), *n.s.* not significant, *OR* Odds ratio, *RR* Relative risk, *qBHs* Quantitative score based on Bradford-Hill criteria (max. 21 points)

[a]Conservative CTS case definition: abnormal nerve conduction findings and symptoms (e. g., paraesthesia, pain, numbness) or clinical signs (positive Phalen's sign or Tinel's sign)

[b]Results refer to American Conference of Governmental Industrial Hygienist (ACGIH) Threshold Limit Value (TLV) for Hand-Activity Level (HAL)

[c]Results refer to eleven studies of high quality with minimised risk of bias

[d]Positive correlation observed

Kozak *et al. BMC Musculoskeletal Disorders* (2015) 16:231

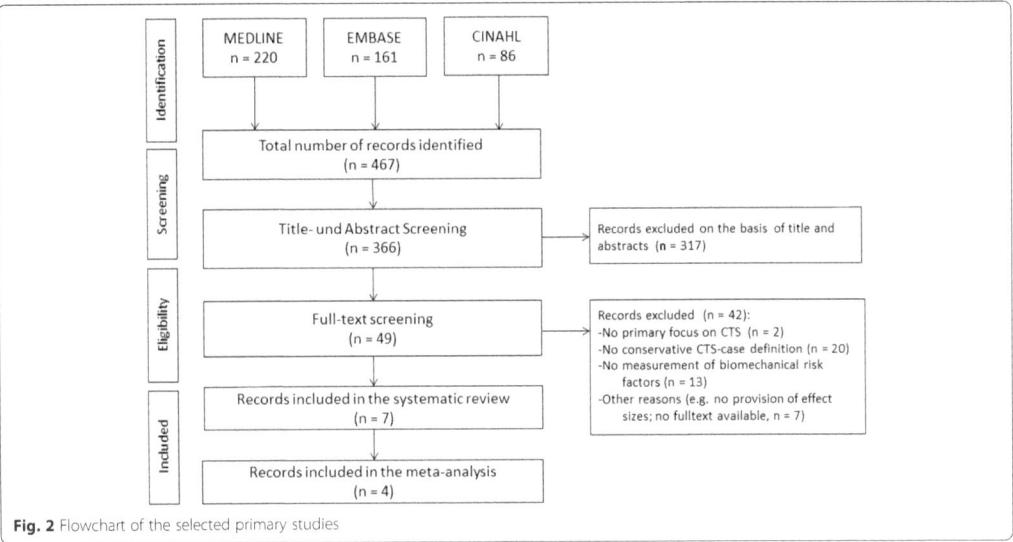

Fig. 2 Flowchart of the selected primary studies

another study with JEM, occupations requiring frequent repetitive motion were significantly associated with CTS, after adjustment for BMI, age and gender. This applied both to the most recent job and to employment duration time-weighted exposures [51]. Two other longitudinal studies showed that repetition in combination with forceful exertion favours CTS [47, 49]. In both case control studies, CTS patients more often reported that they performed repetitive tasks at work than did control groups [52, 53].

Two SRs (grade B) of good quality confirm an association with repetition. Other SRs (*n* = 5) of lower quality do not provide any contradictory results. The findings of all primary studies also confirm this association. Therefore, the quality of evidence for an association between repetition and CTS was upgraded to a high level.

Forceful exertion

Seven SRs (two grade B, three grade C and two grade D) examined the association between force and CTS (Table 3). The two current meta-analyses show that force is positively associated with CTS [31, 41]. However, the study results exhibited significant heterogeneity (I^2 between 84 and 94). Barcenilla et al. [41] showed that most of the heterogeneity could be explained by factors such as CTS case definition, bias risk and the country of the study. The SR conducted by van Rijn et al. [35] confirmed that there is a positive association with CTS in three of seven original studies (consistency: 43 %). Sulsky et al. [44] reported a weak positive association of questionable validity (two of three studies) and Lozano-Calderón et al. [46]

found a weak causal relationship between high force and CTS (Bradford-Hill score: 4.5 of 21 points).

Current primary studies confirm that there is a positive association between force and CTS. At baseline, Burt et al. [48] measured the peak force as the matching value in pounds by dynamometer and expressed as percent of maximum voluntary contraction (% MVC). Workers exposed to a peak force of ≥70 % had a 2.7-fold higher chance of CTS than those with lower levels of peak force (<20 %). Similarly, subjective rating of perceived peak exertion (RPE) on a Borg scale was also positively correlated with a higher probability of CTS (OR 1.14, 95 % CI 1.01–1.29). The longitudinal results show that the percent of time working in forceful exertion had a linear association with CTS. When forceful exertion accounted for more than 20 % of the working time, the risk was increased three-fold; from ≥60 % of the time, the risk was increased 20-fold. Obesity was a significant confounder; when included in the final model, the estimate for forceful exertion increased by 15 % [47]. Garg et al. [49] determined the frequency, intensity and duration of forceful exertion and used this to calculate a Strain Index (SI). At high SI values, the risk of CTS was increased 2.5-fold. Bonfiglioli et al. [50] found that the peak force was a significant predictor of CTS (IRR 1.3, 95 % CI 1.08–1.59). Analysis with JEM confirmed that there is a significant association between forceful motions (dynamic and static strength) at work and the risk of CTS.

Two SRs (grade B) of good quality show a positive association between force and CTS. Other SRs of lower

Publikation 3

Kozak et al. BMC Musculoskeletal Disorders (2015) 16:231

Page 10 of 19

Table 4 Study characteristics and main results of the included primary studies

Author, year	Country	Design	Study population	Outcome	Exposition	Main results from multivariate analyses (95 % Confidence Interval)	Confounder	Quality
Burt et al. 2011 [48]	US	CS (baseline)	n = 464 workers from hospital service[a], engine and bus plant workplaces	Abnormal NCS + symptoms (hand diagram)	ACGIH TLV for HAL; Exertion/min. or time in %)[b]; Peak force (% time)[c]; Flexion/ Extension (% time)[d]; Vibration (observed yes/no)	Peak force ≥20 % vs. <20 %: OR 1.3 (0.6–3.0); peak force ≥70 % vs. <20 %: OR 2.7 (1.3–5.7); exertion ≥15/min vs. <10/min if BMI ≥30: OR 3.4 (1.1–9.9); perceived exertion (unit increase): OR 1.14 (1.0-1.3); ≥AL < TLV vs. <AL: OR 2.3 (0.6-8.9); ≥TLV vs. <AL: OR 3.0 (1.5–5.8); HAL (unit increase) if male: OR 1.4 (1.1–1.8)	Sex; BMI ≥ 30; arthritis; high blood pressure	High (16/20)
Burt et al. 2013 [47]	US	Cohort (2-years)	n = 347 workers from hospital service[a], engine and bus plant workplaces	Abnormal NCS + symptoms (hand diagram)	ACGIH TLV for HAL; TLR; Exertion/min. or time in %)[b]; Peak force (% time)[d]; Flexion/ Extension (% time)[d]; Vibration (observed yes/no)	Exertion/min. ≥20 % vs <20 %: HR 2.8 (1.2–6.8); exertion/min. ≥60 % vs. <20 %: HR 19.6 (6.0–64.2); TLR (unit increase): HR 1.4 (1.1-1.8)	BMI ≥ 30; job strain	High (19/20)
Garg et al. 2012 [49]	US	Cohort (6-years)	n = 551 workers from processing, assembly, manufacturing workplaces	Abnormal NCS + symptoms (intensity ≥25 %/d + duration ≥2 month)	ACGIH TLV for HAL; SI score	≥AL < TLV vs. <AL: HR 1.4 (0.6-3.8); ≥TLV vs. <AL: HR 2.0 (0.8-5.0); SI score >6.1 vs. <6.1: HR 2.5 (1.0-6.1);	Age; BMI ≥ 30; gardening; depression; co-morbidity (other MSDs; arthritis)	High (18/20)
Evanoff et al. 2014 [51]	US	Cohort (3-years)	n = 1107 newly hired workers from construction, technical, laboratory, clerical and hospital service workplaces	Abnormal NCS + symptoms (hand diagram)	Job title based exposure on data from O*NET (job title and requirements): repetitive motion (5-point); static/ dynamic strength (7-point)	Results for most recent jobs (≤6 months): repetitive motion: OR 3.3 (1.4–7.8); static strength: OR 4.4 (1.4–13.9); dynamic strength: OR 3.6 (1.04-12.4);	Age; sex; BMI	Moderate (13/20)
Bonfiglioli et al. 2013 [50]	IT	Cohort (2-years)	n = 2194 workers from factories producing domestic appliances and nursery school	Abnormal NCS + symptoms (hand diagram)	ACGIH TLV for HAL; vibration (observed yes/no)	≥AL < TLV vs. <AL: IRR 2.0 (1.2–3.2); ≥TLV vs. <AL: IRR 2.7 (1.5–4.9); HAL (unit increase): IRR 1.4 (1.2–1.6); peak force (unit increase): IRR 1.3 (1.1–1.6)	Age; sex; BMI; predisposing diseases (0 vs. ≥1)	High (17/20)
Coggon et al. 2013 [53]	GB	CC	n = 475 patients; n = 799 controls	Abnormal NCS + symptoms (duration ≥1 month)	Repeated movements of wrist >4 h/day; repeated bending of elbow >1 h/day; keyboard/ mouse use >4 h/day; vibration >1 h/day	Repeated movements: OR 1.5 (1.1–1.9); vibration: OR 2.4 (1.6–3.8)	Age; sex; BMI; ethnicity; smoking; other diseases; somatic symptoms; mental health; psychosocial factors	Moderate (9/20)

Table 4 Study characteristics and main results of the included primary studies (Continued)

Goodson et al. 2014 [52]	CC	US	n = 87 patients; n = 74 controls	Abnormal NCS + symptoms	Repetition; force; repetition + force combined; vibration; total occupational exposure	Repetition: OR 1.8 (1.5–2.2)	Age, BMI, job satisfaction, vigorous exercise; exercise strain; physical activities	Moderate (12/20)

Abbreviations: *ACGIH* American Conference of Governmental Industrial Hygienists, *AL* Action limit, *BMI* Body mass index, *CC* Case control, *CS* Cross-sectional, *HAL* Hand activity level, *HR* Hazard ratio, *IRR* Incidence rate ratio, *MSD* Musculoskeletal disorders, *NCS* Nerve conduction studies, *O*NET* Occupational Information Network, *OR* Odds ratio, *SI* Strain index score (overall force rating, efforts/min., duration in exertion (%), typical hand/wrist postures; speed of work (h/day)), *TLR* Threshold limit ratio ((Force)/((−0.78)x(HAL) + 7.78)), *TLV* Threshold limit value.

[a]Workers in hospital from central and sterile supply, laboratory, pharmacy, engineering, surgical, kitchen, laundry and administrative support

[b]Exertion per minute were counted from videotape (<10; 10–15; ≥15); percent of time in (forceful) exertion (0–20; 20–60; >60 %)

[c]Force match peak (by dynamometer) represents peak force of job as percent in maximum voluntary contraction MVC/10 (<20 %; 20–70 %; ≥70 %)

[d]Flexion/extension (percent of time spend in range of motion (ROM: 0–20 %; 21–40 %; >40 %)

Kozak *et al. BMC Musculoskeletal Disorders* (2015) 16:231

quality did not provide contradictory results. Four primary studies of high quality confirm the positive association. Thus, the quality of evidence for an association between force and CTS was upgraded to a high level.

Combined exposures (repetition and force)

Two meta-analyses and two SRs (grade B and C, respectively) examined the relationship between CTS and combined exposure patterns (Table 3). Applying the criteria of the National Institute of Occupational Science and Health (NIOSH), Barcenilla et al. [41] found that the risk was doubled, although significant heterogeneity was demonstrated. Subgroup analysis of the studies with a conservative CTS case definition gave borderline significance for a positive association (OR 1.9, 95 % CI 0.99–3.5). In their analyses, Spahn et al. [31] included studies that recorded combined exposure with the ACGIH TLV for HAL score. The authors showed that exposures above TLV were associated with significant increases in the incidence and prevalence of CTS. Two other SRs showed that highly repetitive activities involving forceful exertion increased the risk for CTS in comparison to low exposure [22, 35].

Five current primary studies examined combined exposures (Table 4); four of these had measured the ACGIH TLV for HAL score and were included in the meta-analysis (Figs. 3 and 4) [47–50]. The analysis shows that the risk for CTS is increased at a moderate HAL for TLV (RR 1.5, 95 % CI 1.02–2.31). Values at or above TLV doubled the risk for CTS (RR 2.0, 95 % CI 1.46–2.82). As the studies are homogenous ($I^2 = 0$), no other stratified analyses were performed.

Two SRs (grade B) of high quality with no conflicting results from other SRs support an association between combined exposures and CTS. Findings from four primary studies (meta-analysis) confirm this association. The quality of evidence for an association between combined exposures such as repetition and force was upgraded to a high level.

Vibration

Vibration as risk factor was studied in six SRs (two grade B, three grade C and one grade D). Two current meta-analyses demonstrate an association between exposure to

hand-held vibratory tools and CTS. These results were based on studies with cross-sectional and case control designs [31, 41]. Van Rijn et al. [35] identified three of five original studies (consistency: 60 %) which observed a significant association between vibration and CTS. Sulsky et al. [44] only included a single high-quality study that demonstrated this association. They concluded that the evidence was insufficient. Palmer et al. [22] included six studies in their descriptive analysis and concluded that exposure to hand-held vibratory tools increases the risk of CTS, particularly when tool use is prolonged (>10 years) and/or intensive (>6 h/day). Lozano-Calderón et al. [46] considered that the exposure was a plausible, but debatable risk factor. The Bradford-Hill score was 6.3 of 21 points, which indicates a weak causal relationship.

Five current primary studies examined exposure to vibration, by asking or observing whether employees worked with vibratory tools; no measurements of frequency or intensity (e.g., acceleration) were collected (Table 4) [47, 48, 50–53]. Except for one case control study, vibration was not associated with CTS [53].

Two qualitatively good SRs (grade B) have established an association between vibration and CTS [35, 41]. However, in current high-quality primary studies, vibration was not an independent strong predictor of CTS. Thus, the quality of evidence for an association between vibration and CTS may be classified as moderate.

Wrist posture

Seven SRs have examined the effect of extreme wrist flexion and extension on CTS (Table 3). Barcenilla et al. [41] used the NIOSH criteria and found a positive association (OR 2.7, 95 % CI 1.3–5.5). However, there was significant evidence of heterogeneity, due to differences in CTS case definition and bias risk. In contrast, no association was demonstrated in studies with a conservative CTS case definition (OR 4.7, 95 % CI 0.4–53.3). In the meta-analysis conducted by You et al. [43], exposure was defined as wrist deviation in extension or flexion from neutral wrist posture or duration of time in such postures. They found a two-fold risk of CTS among those who frequently work with non-neutral wrist postures during the workday. After consideration of selection and information bias in subgroup analyses, this

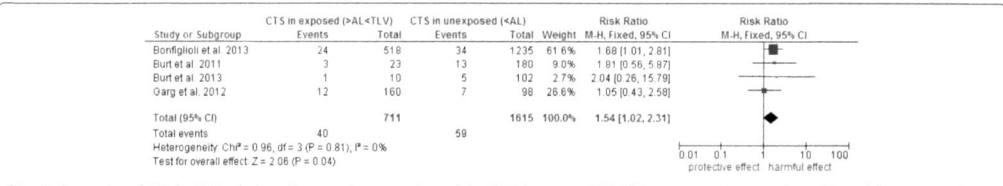

Fig. 3 Forest plot of TLV for HAL – below AL versus between AL and the TLV. Outcome: CTS. Abbreviations: AL, action limit; CI, confidence interval; CTS, carpal tunnel syndrome; HAL, hand activity level; TLV, threshold limit value

Kozak *et al. BMC Musculoskeletal Disorders* (2015) 16:231

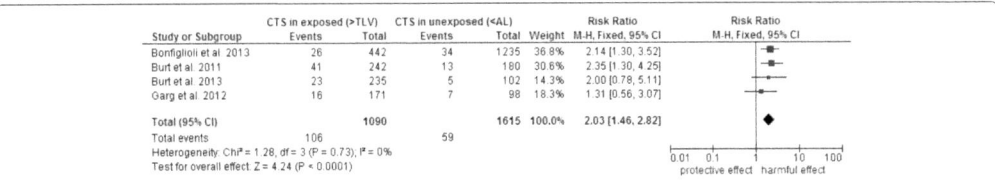

Fig. 4 Forest plot of TLV for HAL – below AL versus TLV and above. Outcome: CTS. Abbreviations: AL, action limit; CI, confidence interval; CTS, carpal tunnel syndrome; HAL, hand activity level; TLV, threshold limit value

effect was confirmed (e.g., only cross-sectional study designs or uniform exposure assessment). However, no subgroup analysis was performed of studies with a conservative CTS case definition. The absence of studies with small sample sizes may indicate publication bias. Another meta-analysis demonstrated an association between chronic flexion posture and CTS (OR 1.7, 95 % CI 1.0–2.6). Significant heterogeneity was present; however, no further subgroup analyses were conducted to resolve heterogeneity [31]. Other SRs found that intensive flexion and extension of the wrist for more than 2 h/day was associated with CTS, particularly in combination with repetition and forceful exertion. Some of the listed studies indicate that there may be a dose-response relationship for the number of hours in these hand positions [22, 35]. In accordance with the Bradford-Hill score, the causality for repetitive hand flexion (5.4 of 21 points) and extension (3.6 of 21 points) was classified as low, with a relatively low consistency (about 40 %) [46].

Some inconsistent results between grade B and C reviews were observed for an association between exposure to non-neutral wrist postures and CTS. Current primary studies did not provide further evidence regarding this relationship. We therefore classified the quality of evidence for an association between non-neutral wrist postures and CTS as low.

Computer use

Two SRs (one grade B and one grade C) which exclusively examined the association between computer use and CTS conclude that there is no evidence for a positive association between computer use and CTS [42, 45]. The results of the meta-analysis demonstrate no association between computer use and CTS (OR 1.7, 95 % CI 0.8–3.6). Moreover, there is no statistically significant association if only the keyboard or mouse use is considered [42]. Other SRs that considered computer use and CTS also failed to find an association (Table 3) [22, 31, 35, 44].

One meta-analysis of good quality (grade B) showed that the epidemiological evidence for a positive association between computer use and CTS is insufficient. Other SRs of lower quality support this finding. Current primary studies do not provide further evidence on this

relationship. Thus, the quality of evidence regarding insufficient association between computer use and CTS was considered moderate.

Discussion

From the epidemiological perspective, this overview and update of the current primary literature confirm that CTS is associated with biomechanical risk factors. High quality of evidence could be established for an association between risk factors such as repetition, forceful exertion, combined exposures and CTS. SRs provide moderate quality of evidence for vibration and low quality of evidence for non-neutral wrist postures. Moderate quality of evidence has been established for an insufficient association between computer use and CTS. Moreover, it has been demonstrated that there is a dose-response relationship between cumulative occupational exposure to force and repetition. A significant increase in risk of CTS was already observed for workers with exposures between AL and the TLV. A further increase in risk was observed for workers with exposures above the TLV.

Consistency of the results

The SRs on the biomechanical factors repetition, forceful exertion and vibration show high consistency and this is confirmed when different occupational groups, methods of measurement and CTS case definitions are considered.

The study results exhibit weak consistency with respect to non-neutral wrist postures and CTS. According to the review on work-relatedness of biomechanical factors, published by the National Institute of Occupational Science and Health (NIOSH) [10], there was insufficient epidemiological evidence that non-neutral wrist postures are an independent risk factor for CTS. However, a causal association has been established in combination with other biomechanical risk factors [10]. Although three current meta-analyses found a two-fold increased risk of CTS, the results are questionable [31, 41, 43]. When considering only studies with a conservative CTS case definition, no significant effect could be found [41]. In the meta-analysis by Spahn et al. [31] an evident heterogeneity was found; however, no further sensitivity analyses were performed to resolve it. One possible

Kozak *et al. BMC Musculoskeletal Disorders* (2015) 16:231

explanation may be the relatively small number of primary studies that examine non-neutral wrist postures as an independent risk factor. Moreover, only a few studies (2 out of 8) employed objective methods of measurement, which could possibly lead to an overestimation of the effect (OR 1.4 versus 3.0) [43]. To deduce reliable exposure levels for flexion and extension, epidemiological studies are required with valid and consistent results for duration and frequency. On the other hand, experimental and clinical studies have found an association between non-neutral wrist postures and CTS. Extreme chronic flexion postures and hyperextension can cause major increases in the carpal tunnel pressure, leading to compression of the N. medianus against the transverse carpal ligament. This can impair the function of the N. medianus – at least in the short term [55].

SRs which studied exposure to computer use came to inconsistent results. An overview of SRs on this association came to the conclusion that there is moderate to high quality of evidence indicating an increased risk of acute pain after intensive use of the mouse or keyboard. However, no evidence was found for the development of specific diseases or chronic pain of the upper extremity [56]. As a complement to Andersen et al.'s [56] overview, we incorporated three additional SRs in our overview, including results from two meta-analyses. These findings provided no further evidence that occupational computer use could lead to relevant increases of CTS [31, 42, 44].

Strength of association
According to the German Social Security Code (SGB VII, § 9, Sentence 8.2), a disease is predominantly of occupational origin if the risk is increased at least two-fold as a consequence of occupational exposure. This corresponds to an aetiological contribution of at least 50 % in exposed workers. With the exception of computer use, risk was increased at least two-fold with all biomechanical factors. Two meta-analyses found that forceful exertion increased the risk by as much as four-fold [31, 50]. Current primary studies confirm that exposure to highly repetitive and forceful exertion resulted in at least a two-fold risk of CTS.

Temporality
A causal relationship is plausible when the exposure to the risk factor occurs prior to the onset of the disease. However, most SRs predominantly included studies with case control or cross-sectional designs, as these require relatively low cost and less time. Lozano-Calderón et al. [46] reported that more than 80 % of the examined studies did not describe the aspect of temporality, which implies that there was a lack of prospective studies. The two SRs of good quality only included three to four prospective studies [35, 41]. Therefore, van Rijn et al. [35] argued that the causality of the observed association had

not been established beyond doubt. However, we included additional primary studies and found a positive temporal association between exposure and CTS [47, 49–51].

As regards the duration of exposure, a pooled analysis of six prospective studies ($n = 3515$; follow-up: 7 years) found that employees who had been working for less than 3.5 years in their current job exhibited a higher incidence rate than those who had had a comparable job for a longer period (HR 3.08, 95 % CI 1.6–6.1) [57]. Another prospective study found that occupations with high repetition and high forceful exertion were associated with increased incidence of CTS after a short occupational exposure of at least 6 months [51]. An exposure period of up to three years can be sufficient to develop occupational CTS. However, the current studies do not allow the conclusion that longer exposure is an argument against a causal association.

Dose–response relationship
On the basis of the SRs, it was not possible to reach a reliable conclusion about a dose-response relationship. By using the ACGIH limits, we demonstrated a statistically significant trend for TLV for HAL and CTS [47–50]. A multiplicative effect is probable, as the risk is greater when two exposure factors are combined [50]. Earlier studies also observed a steady increase in prevalence and incidence of CTS in connection with combined biomechanical loads [58–60]. A current analysis with pooled original data from six prospective studies (mainly from the US) did find a significant increase in risk for exposures above the AL (HR 1.7, 95 % CI 1.2–2.5); however, there was no further increase in risk for those with exposures above the TLV (HR 1.5, 95 % CI 1.0–2.1) [61]. In our meta-analysis we also included a large cohort study on CTS (OCTOPUS cohort) from Italy. Overall, this study attained greater weight than other studies in the analysis and showed a steady increase in risk (Figs. 3 and 4) [50]. The authors conclude, that the current ACGIH limits are not adequate as they might not be sufficiently protective and should therefore be revised [50, 61]. The risk of CTS also increases significantly with an increased amount of time spent in forceful exertion. Burt et al. assume that "force may be the primary job exposure risk factor for CTS" and thus, "a reduction in the amount of time spent in forceful exertion and the intensity of the required force of job tasks may reduce the occurrence of CTS" [47]. It should be mentioned that in the meta-analysis on the ACGIH methods, studies based on observational and direct measurements of force were combined. In the study by Bonfiglioli et al. [50], an experienced ergonomist evaluated the peak force by observing the subjects during their work shifts. The other studies assessed the peak force by using a dynamometer [47–49]. The latter approach is objective, while the other approach depends on the judgement of

Kozak *et al. BMC Musculoskeletal Disorders* (2015) 16:231

the ergonomist. However, the observational method does not imply any inference with the job tasks and does not depend on the workers' behaviour.

Role of confounders

In general, CTS is caused by multiple risk factors. In the general population, CTS is mainly caused by individual risk factors, such as age, gender, obesity and anthropometrics of the hand or other diseases, such as arthritis or diabetes mellitus [62–65]. In contrast to occupational factors, it is comparatively easy to assess individual factors objectively. Nevertheless, a detailed quantitative assessment of the exposure is a major challenge for epidemiological studies, as this must include the frequency, duration and intensity for each activity performed. According to the review based on the Bradford-Hill criteria for causality, the quality and strength of the evidence for a causal association between biological risk factors and CTS were significantly greater than for the occupational risk factors [46]. The authors concluded that, at least at that time, the scientific evidence for occupational risk factors was inadequate and that CTS was largely caused by structural, genetic or biological factors. However, current primary studies with rigorous methods allow the conclusion that occupational risk factors play an important role in the aetiology of CTS. The results of Burt et al. [47, 48] prove that high long-term forceful exertion and repetition are significant independent risk factors for CTS. Obesity (BMI ≥30) is an important confounder. Persons with both individual risk factors such as obesity, as well as occupational risk factors such as high physical demands, have a markedly higher risk of CTS than those with only a single risk factor [48]. It is assumed that the N. medianus is impaired by the fat tissue and/or the swelling in the carpal tunnel [66]. Garg et al. [49] noted that the aetiology of CTS is complex and multifactorial. The combination of repetition and forceful exertion, as measured with the ACGIH TLV for HAL and the Strain Index, was associated with an increased risk of CTS. This was retained after adjustment for essential confounders, such as age, BMI, comorbidities (rheumatoid arthritis and other musculoskeletal diseases of the upper extremities), psychosocial factors and hobbies (gardening). Another prospective study with similar methods also found a significantly increased risk of CTS, after adjustment for known confounders [50].

Limitations of the primary studies in the SRs

In general, there was considerable heterogeneity between the studies with respect to the assessment of the biomechanical risk factors and the outcome definition. Meta-regression analysis showed that the heterogeneity could be significantly explained by differences in the CTS case definitions, study designs, bias scores and

country of study [41]. Differences in CTS diagnostic testing was often mentioned as a limitation in the SRs. Studies with less stringent criteria (e.g., only recording of symptoms) more often found an association, as well as higher values for prevalence and incidence, than did studies with a conservative case definition [46]. Possible consequences might be excessive diagnosis or misclassification of CTS in epidemiological studies [35, 41, 45, 46]. This misclassification is probably differential, as exposed employees may more often suffer symptoms in their hands or fingers than non-exposed participants in the control groups. The combination of a positive nerve conduction test and symptoms or clinical signs gave the most precise results [67]. Barcenilla et al. [41] recommended that a conservative definition of CTS cases should be used in future epidemiological studies. Firstly, this is also used in clinical practice and, secondly, this can probably serve to eliminate a large degree of the studies' heterogeneity.

There has also been criticism that only a few primary studies used objective or direct measurement procedures to assess exposure [22, 35, 41, 43, 46]. For example, van Rijn et al. [35] indicated that the majority of the included studies (66 %) used self-response to quantify the intensity, frequency or duration of exposures. Moreover, different definitions and exposure limits were applied. The lack of adequate statistical power is another limitation and is evident in some studies as wide confidence intervals. Abbas et al. [21] remarked that less rigorous studies tend to employ higher but less precise risk estimates. As the use of a conservative CTS case definition is accompanied by lower prevalence and incidence rates, this must be borne in mind when calculating sample sizes for intended prospective studies.

By including primary studies with a conservative CTS case definition, with objective or direct measurements of exposure and appropriate statistical power, heterogeneity could be avoided in the present meta-analysis and a significant association could be demonstrated between occupational biomechanical risk factors and CTS.

Validity of the included SRs and primary studies

Ultimately, the validity of an overview depends on the validity of the included SRs and primary studies, as well as the processes used for selection and evaluation. One important limitation is that the information we extracted from the SRs has already been filtered and processed by other authors. The reliability of this overview could be greatly influenced by any bias in the review process or by methodological weaknesses in the primary studies included. In an effort to minimise the risk of bias, we prepared this overview in accordance with the PEROSH criteria for SRs and the MOOSE checklist for primary studies. In addition, we excluded narrative reviews, editorials and commentaries a priori.

Kozak *et al. BMC Musculoskeletal Disorders* (2015) 16:231

The methodological validity of the SRs was determined with the AMSTAR-R instrument, which has been found to give a reliable assessment of SRs [32]. Even though the study objectives and outcome were relatively homogenous, the included SRs were of heterogeneous quality. This could be due to differences in the selection and review process, as well as assessment strategy (e.g., study quality and evidence grading). We did not identify any SRs of very good quality (grade A). Only three SRs exhibited good quality (grade B). In general, SRs published within the last five years exhibited higher AMSTAR-R scores which indicates an improvement in the implementation of recommendations for reporting SRs. With one exception [46], the agreement between the reviewers was good to very good (kappa: >0.5). However, items with ambiguous possibilities of interpretation showed a low level of agreement (e.g., Q7: "Was the scientific quality of the included studies assessed and documented?" Q8: "Was the scientific quality used appropriately in formulation conclusions?"). Depending on the research question, SRs of observational studies often used different standards for quality assessment. Although the search strategies or the presentation of the results in the included SRs were relatively consistent, there were considerable differences in the evaluation and interpretation of study quality. There are several checklists and indices for epidemiological studies, particularly observational studies. However, they may differ considerably and do not always fit the planned research question. For this reason, authors sometimes have recourse to a variety of instruments, some of which have not been validated.

In our investigation, the criteria for evaluating the validity of current primary studies were based on publications about similar research questions [35, 36]. This instrument has not been validated, but it covered all essential requirements and was therefore suitable for our purposes. The agreement between the two reviewers was very high: there were no differences in four studies and differences of one to two points in three studies (see Additional file 4). It must be stressed that current primary studies have considered the frequently cited limitations in planning study design. Standardised and objective procedures for testing and measurement are now more frequently used. Statistical power has increased by using larger groups and the period of observation has increased, so that it is now possible to draw conclusions about the temporal link between occupational exposure and outcome.

Quality of evidence

Establishing the quality of evidence for the risk factors employed a qualitative rather than a formal approach and considered the study validity and consistency of the results from SRs and current primary studies. As shown in a descriptive literature analysis of the methodological

implementation of overviews, many authors used the GRADE approach to evaluate the quality of evidence [68]. However, according to Pieper et al. [37], this approach should not be directly transferred to overviews, as some criteria are only suitable for the evaluation of evidence on the basis of primary studies. Overlapping between the study pools is another limitation. In our overview, the overlap rate had the high CCA value of 13.3, i.e., the same references were given in two or more SRs. This led to evidence being counted twice and can considerably restrict its validity. There are currently no formal standardised criteria for this form of summarising evidence. We therefore used a qualitative approach and orientated our study largely towards overviews on musculoskeletal symptoms and diseases, which are also based on epidemiological studies [38, 39, 56]. The postulated core criteria were the validity of the SRs and the consistency of the results. For example, Lakke et al. [39] also considered the validity and consistency of the included cohort studies. Andersen et al. [56] estimated the probability that the observed association is causal. None of these studies carried out an update of current primary literature, so that they were solely dependent on the results of the SRs. Pieper et al. [69] pointed out that the up-to-datedness of the included SRs may be a limitation since new studies may appear during the period between the last literature search and the date of publication. Authors should therefore examine whether including more recent studies may change the conclusion of the review. For this reason, we also included the results of current primary studies in our assessment of the quality of evidence. If there were positive consistent results for biomechanical factors from studies of very high validity, then the quality of the evidence was upgraded. The classification of the degree of evidence into high, moderate, low and poor is not a standardised procedure. This should be borne in mind in the interpretation of the results.

Search and selection process

As we used a validated sensitive search string for aetiological studies, we assume that we had a high detection rate for relevant SRs and primary studies [30]. The inclusion of six languages led to the identification of a meta-analysis in German [31]. A hand search of references and position papers led to the identification of a report from the Occupational Insurance Association for Safety at Work [44]. The search in the Cochrane database gave no relevant hits. The literature search was limited to a specific time frame, thereby making it impossible to exclude publication bias. Furthermore, due to a small number of studies in the meta-analysis, a statistical test or visual assessment of publication bias was not performed.

Kozak *et al. BMC Musculoskeletal Disorders* (2015) 16:231

In order to ensure comparability, the search for primary studies employed the same sensitive search string, with the exception of the partial string for SRs and meta-analyses. One essential inclusion criterion for primary studies was the use of a conservative CTS case definition; this was the most frequent reason for exclusion.

The results were grouped by the exposure factor and this was found to be expedient, as most of the SRs employed this scheme. We also included computer use as an additional exposure factor, as this was considered to be a risk factor in several SRs.

Conclusions

Our study of the available epidemiological results leads us to the conclusion that there is high evidence for an increased risk of CTS in activities requiring a high degree of repetition and forceful exertion. The evidence for vibration is moderate. In current primary studies, exposure to vibration is not a strong independent predictor for CTS. We classified the evidence for an association between non-neutral wrist postures and CTS as low, as the results were inconsistent. It may nevertheless be assumed that, in practice, flexion and extension of the wrist mostly occur in combination with other biomechanical factors. There is no further evidence that CTS is caused by working with a computer keyboard or mouse.

With the exception of computer use, the risk was increased at least two-fold and this indicates that occupational mechanical factors are important independent risk factors for CTS. Short periods of exposure are sufficient for occupational CTS to develop. However, SRs and current primary studies do not permit the conclusion that longer exposure times will lead to a reduction in risk of CTS. A dose-effect relationship between combined exposure and CTS has been demonstrated and even moderate exposures (between AL and TLV for HAL) favour the development of CTS.

To avoid heterogeneity, future aetiological studies on CTS in the occupational setting should employ direct objective measurements of individual activities, with a conservative definition of CTS.

When evaluating the association with occupational biomechanical factors, experts are advised to consider competitive factors such as BMI, age, gender or comorbidities, as they might interact with occupational exposures to some extent. Giersiepen and Spallek [70] point out that a clear delineation from a defined occupational disease is often difficult to determine when several conditions in the same body region are present. However, our synthesis of the latest available evidence suggests that CTS should be considered as an occupational disease after certain biomechanical exposures at the workplace.

Additional files

Additional file 1: A proposed reporting checklist for authors, editors and reviewers of meta-analyses of observational studies in epidemiology (MOOSE). (PDF 24 kb)

Additional file 2: Search terms and strategy used for MEDLINE, EMBASE, CINAHL Databases. (PDF 23 kb)

Additional file 3: Data extraction lists applied separately for systematic reviews and primary studies. (PDF 18 kb)

Additional file 4: Quality assessment criteria applied to primary studies and the quality appraisal **Table S1.** Quality assessment criteria applied to primary studies; **Table S2.** Quality appraisal of the primary studies. (PDF 29 kb)

Additional file 5: Appraisal of systematic reviews using AMSTAR-R tool. (PDF 33 kb)

Competing interests
The authors declare that they have no competing interests.

Authors' contributions
AK participated in the conception of the study, the literature search, data extraction, analysis and interpretation, and was in charge of writing the manuscript. GS participated in developing the study's concept, interpreting data and writing the manuscript. TW participated in the literature search, data extraction and data interpretation. CW participated in the literature search, data extraction and data interpretation. UE participated in the interpretation of the data and contributed to writing the manuscript. AN participated in developing the study's concept, interpreting data and writing the manuscript. All authors read and approved the final manuscript.

Acknowledgements
We thank our colleagues Anja Schablon, Claudia Peters, Dana Wendeler and Peter Koch who provided supplementary information for our overview and meta-analysis. No special funds were received for this study. However, the Institute for Health Services Research in Dermatology and Nursing of the University Medical Centre Hamburg-Eppendorf (UKE) receives an unrestricted fund from the Institute for Statutory Accident Insurance and Prevention in the Health and Welfare Services (BGW) on an annual basis, in order to maintain the research group at the UKE. The funds are provided by a non-profit organisation that is part of the social security system in Germany. The funder had no influence in study design, data collection and analysis, decision to publish, or preparation of the manuscript.

Author details
[1]Institute for Health Services Research in Dermatology and Nursing (CVcare), University Medical Center Hamburg-Eppendorf, Hamburg, Germany. [2]Institution for Statutory Accident Insurance and Prevention in the Health and Welfare Services, Hamburg, Germany. [3]Institute and Policlinic for Occupational and Social Medicine (IPAS), Technical University Dresden, Dresden, Germany.

Received: 6 March 2015 Accepted: 14 August 2015
Published online: 01 September 2015

References
1. Hagberg M, Morgenstern H, Kelsh M. Impact of occupations and job tasks on the prevalence of carpal tunnel syndrome. Scand J Work Environ Health. 1992;18:337–45.
2. Hegmann KT, Thiese MS, Wood EM, Garg A, Kapellusch JM, Foster J, et al. Impacts of differences in epidemiological case definitions on prevalence for upper-extremity musculoskeletal disorders. Hum Factors. 2014;56:191–202.
3. Atroshi I, Gummesson C, Johnsson R, Ornstein E, Ranstam J, Rosen I. Prevalence of carpal tunnel syndrome in a general population. JAMA. 1999;282:153–8.
4. de Krom MC, Knipschild PG, Kester AD, Thijs CT, Boekkooi PF, Spaans F. Carpal tunnel syndrome: prevalence in the general population. J Clin Epidemiol. 1992;45:373–6.

Publikation 3

Kozak *et al. BMC Musculoskeletal Disorders* (2015) 16:231

Page 18 of 19

5. Tanaka S, Wild DK, Seligman PJ, Behrens V, Cameron L, Putz-Anderson V. The US prevalence of self-reported carpal tunnel syndrome: 1988 National Health Interview Survey data. Am J Public Health. 1994;84:1846–8.

6. Salaffi F, De Angelis R, Grassi W. Prevalence of musculoskeletal conditions in an Italian population sample: results of a regional community-based study. I. The MAPPING study. Clin Exp Rheumatol. 2005;23:819–28.

7. Atroshi I, Englund M, Turkiewicz A, Tagil M, Petersson IF. Incidence of physician-diagnosed carpal tunnel syndrome in the general population. Arch Intern Med. 2011;171:943–4.

8. Mondelli M, Giannini F, Giacchi M. Carpal tunnel syndrome incidence in a general population. Neurology. 2002;58:289–94.

9. Aroori S, Spence RA. Carpal tunnel syndrome. Ulster Med J. 2008;77:6–17.

10. Bernard BP. Musculoskeletal disorders and workplace factors – a critical review of epidemiologic evidence for work-related musculoskeletal disorders of the neck, upper extremity, and low back. National Institute of Occupational Safety and Health (NIOSH). 1997. http://www.cdc.gov/niosh/docs/97-141/pdfs/97-141.pdf. Accessed 05 Jun 2014.

11. Palmer KT. Carpal tunnel syndrome: the role of occupational factors. Best Pract Res Clin Rheumatol. 2011;25:15–29.

12. Atcheson SG. Carpal tunnel syndrome: is it work-related? Hosp Pract (1995). 1999;34:49–56.

13. Falkiner S, Myers S. When exactly can carpal tunnel syndrome be considered work-related? ANZ J Surg. 2002;72:204–9.

14. Grabiner MD, Gregor RJ. Revisiting the work-relatedness of carpal tunnel syndrome. Exerc Sport Sci Rev. 2003;31:123–6.

15. Dias JJ, Burke FD, Wildin CJ, Heras-Palou C, Bradley MJ. Carpal tunnel syndrome and work. J Hand Surg (Br). 2004;29:329–33.

16. Stapleton MJ. Occupation and carpal tunnel syndrome. ANZ J Surg. 2006;76:494–6.

17. Thurston A. Aetiology of the so-called 'idiopathic' carpal tunnel syndrome. Curr Orthop. 2000;14:448–56.

18. Nathan PA, Keniston RC, Myers LD, Meadows KD. Longitudinal study of median nerve sensory conduction in industry: relationship to age, gender, hand dominance, occupational hand use, and clinical diagnosis. J Hand Surg [Am]. 1992;17:850–7.

19. Nathan PA, Istvan JA, Meadows KD. A longitudinal study of predictors of research-defined carpal tunnel syndrome in industrial workers: findings at 17 years. J Hand Surg (Br). 2005;30:593–8.

20. Nathan PA, Keniston RC. Carpal tunnel syndrome and its relation to general physical condition. Hand Clin. 1993;9:253–61.

21. Abbas MA, Afifi AA, Zhang ZW, Kraus JF. Meta-analysis of published studies of work-related carpal tunnel syndrome. Int J Occup Environ Health. 1998;4:160–7.

22. Palmer KT, Harris EC, Coggon D. Carpal tunnel syndrome and its relation to occupation: a systematic literature review. Occup Med (Lond). 2007;57:57–66.

23. Becker LA, Oxman AD. Overviews of Reviews, Cochrane Handbook for Systematic Reviews of Interventions. UK: John Wiley & Sons, Ltd; 2008. p. 607–31.

24. Cooper H, Koenka AC. The overview of reviews: unique challenges and opportunities when research syntheses are the principal elements of new integrative scholarship. Am Psychol. 2012;67:446–62.

25. Pieper D, Buechter R, Jerinic P, Eikermann M. Overviews of reviews often have limited rigor: a systematic review. J Clin Epidemiol. 2012;65:1267–73.

26. Pieper D, Antoine SL, Mathes T, Neugebauer EA, Eikermann M. Systematic review finds overlapping reviews were not mentioned in every other overview. J Clin Epidemiol. 2014;67:368–75.

27. Whitlock EP, Lin JS, Chou R, Shekelle P, Robinson KA. Using existing systematic reviews in complex systematic reviews. Ann Intern Med. 2008;148:776–82.

28. OSH Evidence Methods. In: *Clearinghouse of Systematic Reviews*. Partnership for European Research in Occupational Safety and Health (PEROSH). 2012. http://www.perosh.eu/research-projects/perosh-projects/occupational-safety-and-health-evidence-clearinghouse/. Accessed 19 Apr 2014.

29. Stroup DF, Berlin JA, Morton SC, Olkin I, Williamson GD, Rennie D, et al. Meta-analysis of observational studies in epidemiology: a proposal for reporting. Meta-analysis Of Observational Studies In Epidemiology (MOOSE) group. JAMA. 2000;283:2008–12.

30. Mattioli S, Zanardi F, Baldasseroni A, Schaafsma F, Cooke RM, Mancini G, et al. Search strings for the study of putative occupational determinants of disease. Occup Environ Med. 2010;67:436–43.

31. Spahn G, Wollny J, Hartmann B, Schiele R, Hofmann GO. [Metaanalysis for the evaluation of risk factors for carpal tunnel syndrome (CTS) Part II. Occupational risk factors]. Z Orthop Unfall. 2012;150:516–24.

32. Kung J, Chiappelli F, Cajulis OO, Avezova R, Kossan G, Chew L, et al. From systematic reviews to clinical recommendations for evidence-based health care: validation of revised assessment of multiple systematic reviews (R-AMSTAR) for grading of clinical relevance. Open Dent J. 2010;4:84–91.

33. O'Donnell A, Anderson P, Newbury-Birch D, Schulte B, Schmidt C, Reimer J, et al. The impact of brief alcohol interventions in primary healthcare: a systematic review of reviews. Alcohol Alcohol. 2014;49:66–78.

34. Fleiss JL. Statistical methods for rates and proportions. 2nd ed. New York: Wiley; 1981.

35. van Rijn RM, Huisstede BM, Koes BW, Burdorf A. Associations between work-related factors and the carpal tunnel syndrome–a systematic review. Scand J Work Environ Health. 2009;35:19–36.

36. Ariens GA, van Mechelen W, Bongers PM, Bouter LM, van der Wal G. Psychosocial risk factors for neck pain: a systematic review. Am J Ind Med. 2001;39:180–93.

37. Pieper D, Antoine SL, Neugebauer EA, Eikermann M. Up-to-dateness of reviews is often neglected in overviews: a systematic review. J Clin Epidemiol. 2014;67:1302–8.

38. Walton DM, Carroll LJ, Kasch H, Sterling M, Verhagen AP, Macdermid JC, et al. An overview of systematic reviews on prognostic factors in neck pain: results from the international collaboration on neck pain (ICON) project. Open Orthop J. 2013;7:494–505.

39. Lakke SE, Soer R, Takken T, Reneman MF. Risk and prognostic factors for non-specific musculoskeletal pain: a synthesis of evidence from systematic reviews classified into ICF dimensions. Pain. 2009;147:153–64.

40. Deeks JJ, Higgins JPT, Altman DG. Analysing data and undertaking meta-analyses, Cochrane handbook for systematic reviews of interventions. UK: John Wiley & Sons, Ltd; 2008. p. 243–96.

41. Barcenilla A, March LM, Chen JS, Sambrook PN. Carpal tunnel syndrome and its relationship to occupation: a meta-analysis. Rheumatology (Oxford). 2012;51:250–61.

42. Mediouni Z, de Roquemaurel A, Dumontier C, Becour B, Garrabe H, Roquelaure Y, et al. Is carpal tunnel syndrome related to computer exposure at work? A review and meta-analysis. J Occup Environ Med. 2014;56:204–8.

43. You D, Smith AH, Rempel D. Meta-analysis: association between wrist posture and carpal tunnel syndrome among workers. Saf Health Work. 2014;5:27–31.

44. Sulsky SI, Mastroberti MA, Schmidt MD: Quality based critical review of the epidemiological literature on carpal tunnel syndrome and occupation. Hauptverband der gewerblichen Berufsgenossenschaften (HVBG) and Berufsgenossenschaftliches Institut für Arbeitsschutz (BGIA). 2005. http://www.dguv.de/ifa/Publikationen/Reports-Download/BGIA-Reports-2005-bis-2006/BGIA-Report-2-2005/index-2.jsp. Accessed 13 Jun 2014.

45. Thomsen JF, Gerr F, Atroshi I. Carpal tunnel syndrome and the use of computer mouse and keyboard: a systematic review. BMC Musculoskelet Disord. 2008;9:134.

46. Lozano-Calderon S, Anthony S, Ring D. The quality and strength of evidence for etiology: example of carpal tunnel syndrome. J Hand Surg [Am]. 2008;33:525–38.

47. Burt S, Deddens JA, Crombie K, Jin Y, Wurzelbacher S, Ramsey J. A prospective study of carpal tunnel syndrome: workplace and individual risk factors. Occup Environ Med. 2013;70:568–74.

48. Burt S, Crombie K, Jin Y, Wurzelbacher S, Ramsey J, Deddens J. Workplace and individual risk factors for carpal tunnel syndrome. Occup Environ Med. 2011;68:928–33.

49. Garg A, Kapellusch J, Hegmann K, Wertsch J, Merryweather A, Deckow-Schaefer G, et al. The Strain Index (SI) and Threshold Limit Value (TLV) for Hand Activity Level (HAL): risk of carpal tunnel syndrome (CTS) in a prospective cohort. Ergonomics. 2012;55:396–414.

50. Bonfiglioli R, Mattioli S, Armstrong TJ, Graziosi F, Marinelli F, Farioli A, et al. Validation of the ACGIH TLV for hand activity level in the OCTOPUS cohort: a two-year longitudinal study of carpal tunnel syndrome. Scand J Work Environ Health. 2013;39:155–63.

51. Evanoff B, Zeringue A, Franzblau A, Dale AM. Using job-title-based physical exposures from O*NET in an epidemiological study of carpal tunnel syndrome. Hum Factors. 2014;56:166–77.

52. Goodson JT, DeBerard MS, Wheeler AJ, Colledge AL. Occupational and biopsychosocial risk factors for carpal tunnel syndrome. J Occup Environ Med. 2014;56:965–72.

Kozak *et al. BMC Musculoskeletal Disorders* (2015) 16:231

53. Coggon D, Ntani G, Harris EC, Linaker C, Van der Star R, Cooper C, et al. Differences in risk factors for neurophysiologically confirmed carpal tunnel syndrome and illness with similar symptoms but normal median nerve function: a case–control study. BMC Musculoskelet Disord. 2013;14:240.
54. American Conference of Governmental Industrial Hygienists. Threshold Limit Values for chemical substances and physical agents in the work environment. Cincinnati: ACGIH; 2002.
55. Viikari-Juntura E, Silverstein B. Role of physical load factors in carpal tunnel syndrome. Scand J Work Environ Health. 1999;25:163–85.
56. Andersen JH, Fallentin N, Thomsen JF, Mikkelsen S. Risk factors for neck and upper extremity disorders among computers users and the effect of interventions: an overview of systematic reviews. PLoS One. 2011;6:e19691.
57. Harris-Adamson C, Eisen EA, Dale AM, Evanoff B, Hegmann KT, Thiese MS, et al. Personal and workplace psychosocial risk factors for carpal tunnel syndrome: a pooled study cohort. Occup Environ Med. 2013;70:529–37.
58. Silverstein BA, Fine LJ, Armstrong TJ. Occupational factors and carpal tunnel syndrome. Am J Ind Med. 1987;11:343–58.
59. Franzblau A, Armstrong TJ, Werner RA, Ulin SS. A cross-sectional assessment of the ACGIH TLV for hand activity level. J Occup Rehabil. 2005;15:57–67.
60. Violante FS, Armstrong TJ, Fiorentini C, Graziosi F, Risi A, Venturi S, et al. Carpal tunnel syndrome and manual work: a longitudinal study. J Occup Environ Med. 2007;49:1189–96.
61. Kapellusch JM, Gerr FE, Malloy EJ, Garg A, Harris-Adamson C, Bao SS, et al. Exposure-response relationships for the ACGIH threshold limit value for hand-activity level: results from a pooled data study of carpal tunnel syndrome. Scand J Work Environ Health. 2014;40:610–20.
62. Tseng CH, Liao CC, Kuo CM, Sung FC, Hsieh DP, Tsai CH. Medical and non-medical correlates of carpal tunnel syndrome in a Taiwan cohort of one million. Eur J Neurol. 2012;19:91–7.
63. Becker J, Nora DB, Gomes I, Stringari FF, Seitensus R, Panosso JS, et al. An evaluation of gender, obesity, age and diabetes mellitus as risk factors for carpal tunnel syndrome. Clin Neurophysiol. 2002;113:1429–34.
64. Bland JD. The relationship of obesity, age, and carpal tunnel syndrome: more complex than was thought? Muscle Nerve. 2005;32:527–32.
65. Kiani J, Goharifar H, Moghimbeigi A, Azizkhani H. Prevalence and risk factors of five most common upper extremity disorders in diabetics. J Res Health Sci. 2014;14:92–5.
66. Werner RA, Franzblau A, Albers JW, Armstrong TJ. Influence of body mass index and work activity on the prevalence of median mononeuropathy at the wrist. Occup Environ Med. 1997;54:268–71.
67. Rempel D, Evanoff B, Amadio PC, de Krom M, Franklin G, Franzblau A, et al. Consensus criteria for the classification of carpal tunnel syndrome in epidemiologic studies. Am J Public Health. 1998;88:1447–51.
68. Silva V, Grande AJ, Carvalho AP, Martimbianco AL, Riera R. Overview of systematic reviews – a new type of study. Part II Sao Paulo Med J. 2014.
69. Pieper D, Buchter RB, Antoine SL, Eikermann M. [Overviews – status quo, potentials and perspectives]. Z Evid Fortbild Qual Gesundhwes. 2013;107:592–6.
70. Giersiepen K, Spallek M. Carpal tunnel syndrome as an occupational disease. Dtsch Arztebl Int. 2011;108:238–42.

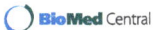

Annals of Work Exposures and Health, 2017, Vol. 61, No. 1, 22–32
doi: 10.1093/annweh/wxw002
Original Articles

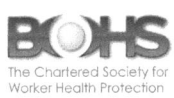
The Chartered Society for
Worker Health Protection

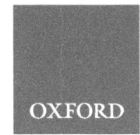
OXFORD

Original Articles

Evaluation of a Training Program to Reduce Stressful Trunk Postures in the Nursing Professions: A Pilot Study

Agnessa Kozak[1]*, Sonja Freitag[2] and Albert Nienhaus[1,2]

[1]Institute for Health Services Research in Dermatology and Nursing, [Center of Excellence for Epidemiology] and Health Services Research for Healthcare Professionals (CVcare), University Medical Center Hamburg-Eppendorf, Martinistraße 52, 20246 Hamburg, Germany; [2]Department for the Principle of Prevention and Rehabilitation, Institution for Statutory Accident Insurance and Prevention in the Health and Welfare Services, Pappelallee 33/35/37, 22089 Hamburg, Germany

*Author to whom correspondence should be addressed. Tel: +49-40-7410-24729; fax: +49-40-7410-59708; e-mail: a.kozak@uke.de

Submitted 9 November 2015; revised 29 August 2016; editiorial decision 1 September 2016; revised version accepted 9 November 2016.

Abstract

Objectives: The aim of this pilot study was to evaluate metrologically the effectiveness of a training program on the reduction of stressful trunk postures in geriatric nursing professions.

Methods: A training program, consisting of instruction on body postures in nursing, practical ergonomic work methods at the bedside or in the bathroom, reorganization of work equipment, and physical exercises, was conducted in 12 wards of 6 nursing homes in Germany. The Computer-Assisted Recording and Long-Term Analysis of Musculoskeletal Loads (CUELA) measurement system was used to evaluate all movements and trunk postures adopted during work before and 6 months after the training program. In total, 23 shifts were measured. All measurements were supported by video recordings. A specific software program (WIDAAN 2.75) was used to synchronize the measurement data and video footage.

Results: The median proportion of time spent in sagittal inclinations at an angle of >20° was significantly reduced (by 29%) 6 months after the intervention [from 35.4% interquartile range (27.6–43.1) to 25.3% (20.7–34.1); $P < 0.001$]. Very pronounced inclinations exceeding 60° [2.5% (1.1–4.6) to 1.0% (0.8–1.7); $P = 0.002$] and static inclinations of over 20° for >4 s [4.4% (3.0–6.7) to 3.6% (2.5–4.5); $P < 0.001$] were significantly reduced, by 60% and 22%, respectively. Video analysis showed that in 49% of care situations, ergonomic measures were implemented properly, either at the bedside or in the bathroom.

Conclusions: Stressful trunk postures could be significantly reduced by raising awareness of the physical strains that frequently occur during a shift, by changes in work practices and by redesigning the work environment. Workplace interventions aimed at preventing or reducing low back pain in nursing personnel would probably benefit from sensitizing employees to their postures during work.

Keywords: bending; ergonomics; geriatric nurses; metrological evaluation; musculoskeletal disorders; stressful trunk posture; training program

Introduction

Although low back pain (LBP) is common among the working-age population and the causes are multifactorial (Balague *et al.*, 2012), nursing personnel are more likely to suffer from LBP than the general population. A recent review found that the 12-month mean prevalence of LBP in nursing personnel is 55% (Davis and Kotowski, 2015). A review of the global prevalence of LBP in the general population reported a lower mean prevalence of 38% (Hoy *et al.*, 2012). The development of LBP is attributed to the frequency of transfers (Engkvist *et al.*, 2000; Holtermann *et al.*, 2013), as well as the repositioning and handling of patients (Smedley *et al.*, 1995; Eriksen *et al.*, 2004). A recent review of the work relatedness of LBP in nursing personnel found convincing evidence of a causal relationship between the mechanical stress caused by patient-handling activities and LBP. However, other patient care tasks—such as bathing, dressing, or feeding—are also associated with an elevated risk and confound the dose–response assessment of patient lifting alone (Yassi and Lockhart, 2013).

Interventions to reduce or prevent physical workload and LBP in nursing have been studied for many years and mainly focus on training in manual patient handling (Videman *et al.*, 1989; Best, 1997), exercise training (Dehlin *et al.*, 1981; Gundewall *et al.*, 1993), stress reduction training (Horneij *et al.*, 2001), or multidimensional strategies (Garg and Owen, 1992; Alexandre *et al.*, 2001). Four systematic reviews have evaluated the effect of interventions on prevention or reduction of LBP and injuries in health professions and demonstrate moderate level of evidence for multidimensional intervention strategies (e.g. education and training combined with an ergonomic intervention). However, they found high evidence that interventions based solely on training in patient handling had no effect on LBP (Hignett, 2003; Bos *et al.*, 2006; Dawson *et al.*, 2007; Tullar *et al.*, 2010). Since training in manual handling alone—which has been the principle focus of workplace interventions—is unlikely to be successful in reducing musculoskeletal disorders (MSD), other work-related aspects need to be taken into account.

Although lifting and transferring patients impose high strains on the spine, nurses spend only a short time on these tasks during the course of a working day. Hodder *et al.* (2010) found that patient care tasks (e.g. bathing, dressing, and feeding) and miscellaneous tasks (e.g. making beds) account for almost 50% of shift duration, while lifting accounted for only 4%. Similarly, Freitag *et al.* (2007) found that, on average, 2 min per shift were spent transferring patients. To perform patient and non-patient care activities, nurses frequently had to bend forward or work for extended periods in a static trunk inclination. Repeated bending and awkward trunk postures are under consideration as additional risk factors for the development of LBP, as they increase the exertion and muscle power required to complete a task (Occupational Safety and Health Administration, 2009). To our knowledge, only a few intervention studies have focussed on postural alignment (Engels *et al.*, 1998; Pohjonen *et al.*, 1998; Fanello *et al.*, 1999; Nussbaum and Torres, 2001). Compared to controls, they found a significant increase in upright/safe postures and fewer errors after ergonomic educational training.

In a prior study in geriatric wards, we found that sagittal inclinations exceeding an angle of 60° were most often triggered by bed making (22%), clearing up/cleaning (16%), and basic care activities (16%) (Freitag *et al.*, 2007). In a subsequent experimental study, we examined the influence of different bed heights (knee, thigh, and hip) and work methods in the bathroom (standing, kneeling, and sitting) on forward-bending postures. The proportion of time spent in an upright position increased significantly, by almost 20%, when the bed was raised from thigh to hip height. Similarly, working in a sitting, rather than a standing, position in the bathroom resulted in a significant increase (26%) in the time spent in an upright position (Freitag *et al.*, 2014).

Taking the preliminary findings into account, the objective of the present study was to conduct and evaluate the effectiveness of a training program aimed at reducing stressful trunk postures in geriatric nurses, by raising their awareness of frequent bending occurring during specific care tasks and procedures. Moreover, the training program also included instructions in practical ergonomic work at the bedside and in the bathroom, as well as ergonomic reorganization of working materials and redesign of residents' room.

Methods

Study procedure and population

A convenience sample of six facilities, each with two wards, took part. Two voluntary participants were recruited from each participating ward. They were measured using the personal Computer-assisted Recording and Long-term Analysis of Musculoskeletal Loads (CUELA) measuring system throughout an early shift, before and after the intervention. The first measurement was conducted 2 weeks before the start of the intervention, and the same subjects were measured again 6 months later. In order to minimize disruption of the regular ward routine during measurement, only one measuring system per ward and early shift was used. Two measuring systems were used in parallel in the two wards of the respective facility. The measurements were taken on two consecutive days.

There were several conditions for inclusion in the study. During the study phase, the institutions had to have exclusively height-adjustable beds, and they were not to be planning any alterations, certifications, mergers, or other research projects during this period. Participants who wore the CUELA measuring system had to be prepared to take part in the training activities. They had to be female, without a senior management position, and not trainees. Moreover, the participants had to be available for at least three-quarters of a year (i.e. they had no intention to resign or change jobs and were not pregnant or planning any lengthy in-service training or leave of absence). Participants had no back problems that might have inhibited their performance of specific care tasks. Furthermore, all employees and managers of the participating wards had to attend the basic seminar.

A total of 23 early shifts (T_0) were measured and recorded. During the second measurement, we identified measurement uncertainties attributable to the CUELA system in three participants. Measurement of another participant had to be terminated prematurely for personal reasons. We therefore obtained complete measurement data (T_1) for 19 participants.

In the participating facilities, all participating employees, residents, and their relatives were given detailed information about the study goals and programs (e.g. measuring system, video filming) in advance, and consent forms were obtained for participation and for videos and photos to be taken. This study was approved by the Ethics Committee of the Hamburg Medical Association (Ärztekammer Hamburg, Germany).

Contents of the intervention program

To reduce stressful trunk postures, we designed a 2-day basic seminar and two follow-up training sessions. In each facility, intervention began with a basic seminar in which not only the test participants but also all employees of the two participating wards were involved. In order to maintain regular operations in the wards, the seminar was held twice in each facility, with half the employees from each of the two wards participating on each occasion. The basic seminar focused on the theory of body postures in the care professions, on body awareness training and physical exercises, on setting/equipment modifications, and on practical ergonomic work methods at the bedside and in the bathroom. In a participatory ergonomic intervention, we began by describing and discussing the occupational risks of musculoskeletal MSD in the care profession. Pictorial material was then used to sensitize participants to the body postures that they frequently adopted during a work shift. The corresponding work situations were then analysed interactively, and alternative ergonomic solutions were discussed. The aforementioned laboratory study not only showed that raising the bed height and using a stool in the bathroom led to a reduction in unfavourable body postures but also that when participants adhered to these ergonomic principles they felt that their work was less stressful (Freitag et al., 2014). These findings were taken into account in practical implementation of ergonomic ways of working at the residents' bedsides and in the bathroom (Table 1).

Eight weeks after the basic seminar, we held a half-day follow-up training session, followed by another 12 weeks later. These follow-up training sessions were offered only to test participants and took the form of advice and support during an early shift. Two weeks after the basic seminar, we conducted a telephone interview with the participants. This was followed by a second telephone interview 2 weeks after the first follow-up training session. Respondents were asked to report the extent to which they were implementing the seminar contents in their daily work. Those who had difficulties with implementation were asked about the underlying reasons. For this purpose, we used a standardized interview guide with 18 closed or open questions. Open questions were analysed by frequency of citation (see Supplementary Table 1 is available at *Annals of Work Exposures and Health* online).

Questionnaire

A questionnaire was used to establish the following variables for participants: age, weight, height, professional experience (in years), type of training (geriatric nurse, hospital nurse, or geriatric or nursing care assistant), occupational status (no leading position, deputy ward manager, ward manager), scope of employment (full time or part-time), general state of health (five-point Likert scale), work ability (five-point Likert scale), and whether they had any illness or injury that impeded their

Annals of Work Exposures and Health, 2017, Vol. 61, No. 1

Table 1. Contents of the intervention program.

Knowledge transfer on body postures in nursing professions

Information on physical strains in nursing care and the associated risks to the musculoskeletal system, with the focus on the spine

Ergonomic findings from previous studies in nursing care

Body awareness training and physical exercises

Body postures at work (e.g. to sensitize participants to the body postures adopted while working, photographs of actual care situations were shown, and body postures in the corresponding work situation were discussed)

Body strength and coordination training (e.g. to raise participants' awareness of their own body tension and posture, various exercises were taught on coordination and body tension)

Physical exercises (e.g. to strengthen and relax the spine muscles, exercises that can be carried out during routine work were demonstrated)

Ergonomic practical instructions

Basic care activities were carried out at a typical resident's bedside and in the bathroom. The aim was for participants to draw a direct comparison and sense for themselves just how much working with a raised bed or sitting on a stool relieves strain

Every participant was asked to perform activities twice in succession: (i) first at a low bed (thigh height) and then with the bed at the optimal (hip) height, (ii) first in a standing or kneeling position and then sitting on a stool in the resident's bathroom

Reorganization and redesign

Reorganization of working materials and ergonomic redesign of the resident's room (e.g. frequently used utensils or clothing were re-sorted and placed at an ergonomic height)

Use of a care basket for stowing care utensils in daily use. This is intended to prevent repeated bending forward to the bedside cupboard

Use of a laundry basket to reduce repeated bending to pick up dirty laundry from the floor

work performance. We subsequently calculated body mass index from the weight and height variables.

While the measurements were being taken, the ward managers of the 12 participating wards were questioned about the following aspects: number of (height-adjustable) beds and current occupancy, number of qualified and non-qualified care workers on the early shift, and availability of aids (e.g. lifters, sliding mats, transfer boards). A nurse-to-resident staffing ratio was calculated by dividing the number of occupied beds per ward by the number of nurses on the early shift.

Measurement system and video recordings

The CUELA measurement system and video analyses were used to evaluate this intervention. CUELA has been demonstrated to have good validity and reliability in laboratory investigations and field studies (Berufsgenossenschaftliches Institut für Arbeitsschutz, 1998; Ellegast *et al.*, 2009). Figure 1 shows the measuring system in use on a geriatric care ward. Sensors on the thoracic and lumbar spine recorded data on locational and angular positions at a frequency of 50 Hz. This permits accurate kinematic reconstruction of the subject's movements. The participants were able to move freely without restrictions since they were not connected to any external components. They were instructed to carry out their work as usual. The measuring system was only switched off during breaks, documentation,

or handover interviews, since these work tasks are normally performed while sitting. For each measurement, participants were filmed throughout the shift. Specially developed software (WIDAAN 2.79) was used to synchronize the measurement data and video footage. Thus, it allowed precise allocation of the measurement data to each work task performed by the nurse during the shift. For accurate synchronization of real-work situations, an animated computer figure represented the corresponding measured values (Freitag *et al.*, 2007, 2012).

Care intensity score

The intensity of care for individual residents and thus the basic care required (e.g. bed making, washing, or dressing) varies considerably. In order to take this into account, in a preliminary study, we developed a basic care intensity score (Freitag *et al.*, 2012). This score was assessed for both time points, in order to examine whether intensity of care differed or remained constant over time. The number of residents a nurse had to care for while measurements were being taken was ascertained by video analyses. Each resident was allocated a number of points corresponding to the effort expended (1 = nurse only made the bed; 2 = nurse made the bed and <50% of basic care activities; 3 = nurse made the bed and >50% of basic care activities). This figure was added to the total points for the particular shift. The higher the total score per nurse, the higher the intensity of care provided to residents (Freitag *et al.*, 2012).

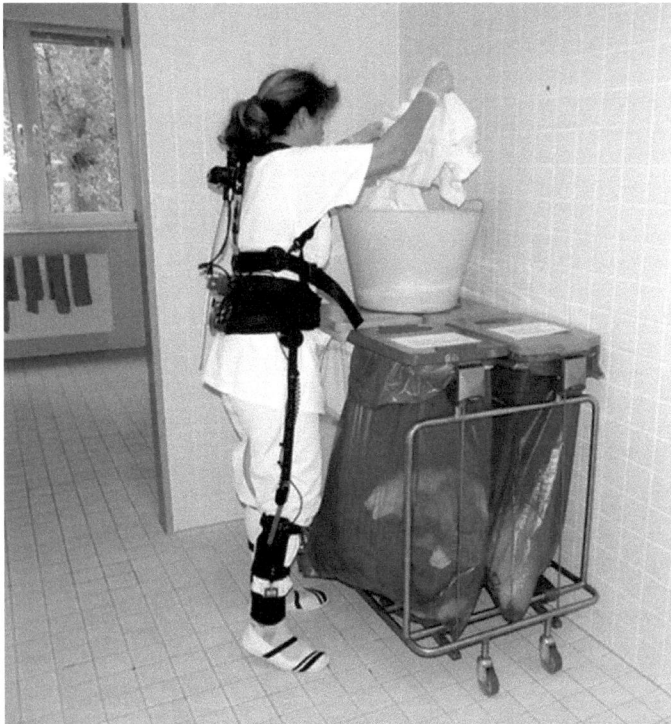

Figure 1. A nurse is wearing the CUELA measurement system while working. Sensors on the thoracic and lumbar spine deliver three-dimensional data on trunk movements.

Trunk postures and video analysis

According to ISO 11226 (ISO, 2000) and DIN EN 1005-4 (DIN, 2005), sagittal inclinations between 0° and 20° are within the acceptable range and are designated as upright postures. Pressure on the spinal disk is lowest in this position. It increases in line with increasing sagittal inclination (Wilke *et al.*, 1999). Sagittal inclinations between 20° und 60° are classified as conditionally acceptable and of >60° as unacceptable (ISO, 2000; DIN, 2005). According to DIN EN 1005-1 standard (DIN, 2002), trunk postures that were maintained for >4 s at a constant or slightly changing force were defined as static postures. We calculated the frequency and the proportion of the work shift spent in those postures. The functioning of the measuring system and the ergonomic evaluation of body postures in a care setting have been described in detail in earlier publications (Freitag *et al.*, 2007, 2012).

The video recordings made during the follow-up measurements were evaluated by a skilled observer, who began by identifying the number of care situations for each participant at the bedside and in the bathroom. The observer then assessed whether the participant implemented the proper measures at the bedside (raising the bed to hip height) and in the bathroom (using a stool). If the bed was raised to thigh height only, the observer rated the measure as having been partially implemented. However, in few basic care situations, the residents requested us to switch off the camera for privacy reasons.

Statistical analyses

The metric variables were expressed as a mean with standard deviations or median with interquartile range; categorical data were presented as counts (percentages). Differences between two measurements were assessed by using a paired-samples *t*-test and, as a non-parametric alternative, a Wilcoxon matched pair signed-rank test. Hodges–Lehman estimates for the differences between two samples with a 95% confidence interval were presented. In addition, we calculated the relative change between the two measurements $[(T_1 - T_0)/T_0] \times 100$. *P*-values of <0.05, two-tailed, were considered statistically significant. Analyses were performed with IBM SPSS Version 22.0.

Annals of Work Exposures and Health, 2017, Vol. 61, No. 1

Results

Measurement data were available from 23 participants at baseline and from 19 participants at a 6-month follow-up. After a short adjustment period, participants became accustomed to the system while performing daily tasks; no restrictions on functionality and performance were reported. The mean measurement time per shift was similar at baseline and follow-up (326 and 315 min, respectively). All 12 wards were almost fully occupied and equipped with ergonomic aids and height-adjustable beds. A nurse-to-resident ratio of 1:8 showed that on average one nurse cared for eight residents per shift. The mean basic care intensity score was nearly identical for the two time points (21 points), though more residents were in need of intensive care (Stage 3) (Table 2). The participants had worked an average of 17 (± 8.7) years in the care sector. Almost two-thirds worked part-time, were registered nurses, or held no leading position. The majority rated their health as good or very good. Impairment due to disease or injury was reported by five participants (22%), but only one person had some restrictions during work. Twenty-two percent rated their work ability as fair. Further participant characteristics are shown in Table 3.

After the intervention, the median proportion of time spent in sagittal inclinations exceeding 20° was significantly reduced, by 29% ($P < 0.001$), from 1772 to 1708 median trunk movements per shift. The proportion of very pronounced inclinations exceeding 60° was reduced by 60% ($P = 0.002$), from 288 to 135 inclinations per shift. A significant reduction in static inclinations was also detected (22%; $P < 0.001$), from 462 to 329 inclina-

tions per shift (numbers of inclinations not in the table). The median time spent in sagittal inclinations exceeding 20° was reduced by 27 min per shift (Table 4).

Results of the video analyses at the second measurement show that in total 217 basic care activities at the bedside were observed. As recommended by the seminar instructor, the bed was raised to hip height in 44.7% of all care situations. However, in 44.2% of situations, the bed was partially raised, and in 11.1%, the bed was not raised at all. In total, 52 care situations in the bathroom were observed. A stool was used in 67.3% of these situations to perform basic care in the sitting position; in 32.7% of the situations, the stool was not used by the nurses (Table 5).

Supplementary Table 1 available at *Annals of Work Exposures and Health* online shows the main results of the first telephone interviews 2 weeks after the seminar. Participation rate in the first interview was 96% ($N = 22$) and in the second interview 57% ($N = 13$). Since there were no relevant differences in responses between the first and second interviews, we analysed information gained from the first telephone interview on account of the high participant rate. All participants reported that they were more conscious of adopting awkward postures during work. The majority (96%) paid more attention to raising beds to an ergonomic height. However, 50% admitted to not having adjusted the bed properly in some stressful working situations. The majority (91%) reported that they had performed some bedside tasks differently (e.g. using ergonomic mobilization techniques) or had reorganized residents' wardrobes or drawers (e.g. placing frequently used laundry or equipment at an ergonomic

Table 2. Ward- and care-related factors.

Ward-related factors ($N = 12$ wards)	Proportions (95% CI)
Residents per nurse and per shift (n)	8.1 (7.2–9.0)
Occupancy rate	96% (93%–97.4%)
Rate of height-adjustable beds	100% (72%–100%)
Rate of wards equipped with ergonomic aids[a]	92% (63%–100%)
Rate of registered geriatric nurses per shift	50% (35%–65%)
Care-related factors ($N_{T0} = 23$ participants)	Mean (± SD)
Basic care intensity score (points)	T_0 21.0 (± 4.8); T_1 21.6 (± 6.4)[b]
Number of patients provided with basic care—Stage 1[c]	T_0 1.1 (± 1.1); T_1 1.3 (± 1.4)[b]
Number of patients provided with basic care—Stage 2[d]	T_0 0.6 (± 0.8); T_1 0.5 (± 0.8)[b]
Number of patients provided with basic care—Stage 3[e]	T_0 6.2 (± 1.5); T_1 6.5 (± 2.0)[b]

CI, confidence interval; SD, standard deviation.
[a]Gliding boards, lifters.
[b]Statistically not significant.
[c]Stage 1—making beds; no other basic care tasks.
[d]Stage 2—making beds and <50% of other basic care tasks.
[e]Stage 3—making beds and >50% of other basic care tasks.

Table 3. Characteristics of the participants (N_{70} = 22[a]).

Demographic and work-related factors	N (%) or mean (± SD)
Age (years)	
≤39	4 (17.3)
≤49	11 (47.8)
≤59	7 (39.1)
Height (cm)	167 (± 7.6)
BMI	23.4 (± 3.1)
Professional experience (years)	17 (± 8.7)
Part-time employment	14 (60.9)
Educational background	
Registered (geriatric) nurse	14 (60.9)
Nursing assistant	8 (34.8)
Managerial position	
No leading position	15 (65.2)
Group or deputy ward manager	7 (30.3)
Health-related factors	
Health status	
Excellent or very good	8 (34.8)
Good	11 (47.8)
Less well	2 (8.7)
Impairment due to disease or injury	
No impairment	16 (69.6)
Complaints but no restrictions during work	4 (17.4)
Complaints and some restrictions during work	1 (4.3)
Work ability (regarding physical strain)	
Excellent	6 (26.1)
Quite or very good	10 (43.5)
Fair	5 (21.7)

BMI, body mass index; SD, standard deviation.

[a]Complete information for one case was missing; information on health-related factors was missing for another case.

height). To avoid frequent bending, they also used a care basket for daily care utensils (100%), a laundry basket (64%), and a stool during care activities in the bathroom (64%). Only a few participants (14%) encountered some problems when implementing these measures. The main reasons were time pressure due to understaffing, other priorities, or residents requesting otherwise.

Discussion

In this metrological evaluation, we found that frequent bending by geriatric nursing staff could be significantly reduced by means of participatory ergonomics, body and posture awareness training, and physical training. The time spent in sagittal inclinations of >20° was signifi-

cantly reduced, from ~2 to 1.5 h per shift, 6 months after training. Video analyses showed that in 49% of the care situations, ergonomic measures were implemented as recommended, either at the bedside or in the bathroom. These observations suggest that there is considerable additional potential to further reduce frequent bending. Overall, the participating nurses judged the scope and content of the training as helpful and appropriate. One should bear in mind, however, that our training program was not aimed primarily at reducing LBP but at increasing overall awareness of body postures and physical strains that nursing staff hardly notice during their work.

In line with our previous findings, at baseline, the geriatric nurses spent 36% of the measured time in a forward-bending position (Freitag et al., 2012). However, results of continuous posture monitoring studies in geriatric nurses showed that less time was spent in flexed postures (Jansen et al., 2001; Hodder et al., 2010; Ribeiro et al., 2011). By using an inclinometer, Jansen et al. (2001) showed that geriatric nurses spent ~21% of their working time at an angle of >20°, and in the study by Hodder et al. (2010), the participants spent 25% of their time at an angle of >30°. Using the Spineangle accelerometer, Ribeiro et al. (2011) showed that 5% of work time was spent in flexed postures at an angle of >30°. These substantial differences were mainly the result of the different devices used and the location in which they were attached to the body. While we measured the mean inclination of the entire trunk, Jansen et al. (2001) and Ribeiro et al. (2011) measured the inclination of the lumbar spine and Hodder et al. (2010) measured the inclination of the thoracic spine.

When monitoring trunk postures during work, it should be noted that 19% of all non-neutral inclinations are coupled with lateral and/or torsional movement of the trunk (Freitag et al., 2007). However, we evaluated the sagittal inclinations of the trunk, as these movements are associated with increased intradiscal pressure, resulting in greater spine loads than twisting or lateral bending (Nachemson, 1975). As in our previous study, we detected a large number of static postures per shift (Freitag et al., 2012). After training, these were significantly reduced by 22%. Nurses themselves reported static postures as one of the main physical stressors at work (Engels et al., 1996). In a study involving a course in ergonomic education, a decreasing trend in awkward postures and errors while performing nursing tasks was observed in the group receiving this intervention (Engels et al., 1998).

After being made aware of the repeated bending during a shift and the actual time needed to raise a bed, the majority of participants in the present study

Annals of Work Exposures and Health, 2017, Vol. 61, No. 1

Table 4. Time spent in different trunk postures before and after the intervention.

Inclinations	Mdn$_{baseline}$ (IQR)	Mdn$_{follow-up}$ (IQR)	Hodges–Lehman estimates (95% CI)	RC (%)	*P* value
Proportion of SI ≥ 20° (%)	35.4 (27.6–43.1)	25.3 (20.7–34.1)	–7.7 (–11.1 to –4.3)	–29	<0.001
Proportion of SI ≥ 60° (%)	2.5 (1.1–4.6)	1.0 (0.8–1.7)	–1.3 (–3.2 to –0.5)	–60	0.002
Proportion of static SI ≥ 20° for >4 s (%)	4.4 (3.0–6.7)	3.6 (2.5–4.5)	–1.4 (–2.3 to –0.6)	–22	<0.001
Duration of SI ≥ 20° (min)	104 (90–134)	77 (66–103)	–27.3 (–40.5 to –15.5)	–26	<0.001

CI, confidence interval; IQR, interquartile range; Mdn, median; RC, relative change [($T_1 - T_0$)/T_0] × 100; SI, sagittal inclinations.

Table 5. Implementation rates of work methods at the bedside and in the bathroom.

Location	Care situations per shift and nurse	Measure implemented correctly	Measure partly implemented	Measure not implemented
	N	*n* (%)	*n* (%)	*n* (%)
At the bedside	217	97 (44.7)	96 (44.2)	24 (11.1)
In the bathroom	52	35 (67.3)	—	17 (32.7)
Total	269	132 (49)	137 (51)	

reported that they paid more attention to raising beds to an ergonomic height. However, one-half also reported situations where they did not raise a bed appropriately. They frequently explained this with stress or time pressure (Supplementary Table 1 is available at *Annals of Work Exposures and Health* online). This coincides with the video analyses, in which we found that in 55% of bedside care situations, nurses only partially raised the bed, if at all. Although proper adjustment of the resident's bed resulted in better working postures and less strain on the body (Freitag *et al.*, 2014), nurses argued that this procedure was time consuming (Petzäll *et al.*, 2001). However, it takes an average of 53–59 s to raise a bed from knee to hip height (Freitag *et al.*, 2014). One further reason why nurses often failed to adjust beds to hip height could be a lack of awareness of how often they bend their trunk forward during a shift (Freitag *et al.*, 2007, 2012). As regards the use of stools during personal care, we found that more than two-thirds of nurses performed basic care in the sitting position. This was confirmed by the interviews (64%). Although we did not ask for impediments, we assume that a lack of space for manoeuvre in residents' bathrooms might be one reason. Another possible explanation is that nurses are not accustomed to perform basic care in a sitting position.

Several studies have shown that nurses spend a high proportion of time in non-patient-handling tasks dur-ing a shift (Engels *et al.*, 1994; Freitag *et al.*, 2007; Hodder *et al.*, 2010; Holmes *et al.*, 2010). Merely focusing on patient-handling tasks such as lifting or repositioning may therefore lead to an underestimation of the overall strain in nursing. As regards the relationship between occupational postural exposure such as frequent or sustained flexion and the development of LBP, conflicting evidence has been reported (Bakker *et al.*, 2009; Ribeiro *et al.*, 2012). Systematic reviews using Bradford–Hill criteria for causality conclude that occupational bending/twisting and awkward postures are not independently causative of LBP (Roffey *et al.*, 2010; Wai *et al.*, 2010). Body posture may lead to excessive biomechanical stress on the musculoskeletal system, although epidemiological studies suggest that the role of body posture on the development of LBP is debatable (Solomonow *et al.*, 2003; Olson *et al.*, 2004; Solomonow, 2004). Wai *et al.* (2010) suggested that differences in the outcome and postural measurement approaches may lead to inconsistent results for this relationship. Nonetheless, several studies on nursing professions reported a positive association between postural exposure and LBP (Josephson *et al.*, 1998; Jansen *et al.*, 2004; Yip, 2004). According to Holtermann *et al.* (2013), frequent lifting and carrying of a low load mass with the back bent forward doubled the risk of chronic LBP in female nursing staff, whereas lifting and carrying any load mass with an upright back did not increase the risk.

The advantage of our study was the use of the CUELA measurement system coupled with video recordings to evaluate the effectiveness of the training program. As no external connection to system components was required and the weight of the equipment was reasonable (2.7 kg), the nurses could move freely and without limitation in performing their daily care routine. The WIDAAN specially developed software synchronized the measurement data and video recordings, so that each trunk posture could be assigned to the corresponding work situation.

Several limitations should be pointed out. When we set out to implement and evaluate the training program in body postures in geriatric care facilities, we faced some acquisition problems. Facilities refused to participate in this study—mainly because their daily routine had to be filmed while measurements were taken. There may therefore be a selection bias that might affect the generalizability of the study results. Although residents had given their consent to video recordings, in few basic care situations, we were asked to switch off the camera for privacy reasons. Thus, the proportion of the care activities might have been underestimated. As the video footage might not display the complete working tasks, the evaluation of the effectiveness could show some inaccuracies.

Another drawback arises from the observation bias, also known as the Hawthorne effect. As the participants had to wear the measurement system and were filmed while working, it is likely that they automatically changed their behaviour to fit the expected results. Hence, our results may considerably underestimate the frequency and duration of sagittal inclination. In the previous CUELA study, the nurses also reported that patients made an unusual effort to cooperate with them during the course of measurement (Freitag et al., 2012).

Implementation of the CUELA system made high logistical demands on participating facilities and the research team. Therefore, only two voluntary participants from the two wards in each facility were measured and videotaped during work. As a result, the sample size was rather small. In addition, the focus in this work-site intervention was on relatively short-term training effects rather than on potential prevention or reduction of LBP injury. The sustainability of such ergonomic training is therefore doubtful and has to be explored in further studies investigating health-related outcomes with frequent refresher units and at least a 1-year follow-up.

Furthermore, results from pre-experimental designs (without a control group) should be interpreted with caution, since they pose a threat to the internal validity.

To examine the significance of the behavioural change due to the training program, a randomly selected control group should be considered to reduce the effect of known or expected sources of variability, and thus to improve the precision of our results, to exclude alternative explanations, and to establish a causal relationship. However, the study presented here pursues an exploratory approach to establish whether the observed effect is worthy of further investigation. The effectiveness of this training concept should be investigated by a randomized controlled trial with extended follow-up periods. On the basis of the results of this study, we estimated that with a power of 90%, 12 wards with three individuals per ward would be sufficient for a proper cluster randomized controlled trial to validate the effects.

In this evaluation, we did not quantify the effects of force on the spine. Future studies should consider continuous posture monitoring to evaluate low back loads. Holmes et al. (2010) used an inclinometer to evaluate peak and cumulative lumbar spine loads in long-term care nurses. Eighty percent of cumulative compression originated from activities such as personal care, unloaded standing, walking, or other activities, whereas 10% resulted from lifting and transferring patients. Although transfers and lifts contributed to high peak loads, little time was spent on those tasks (Holmes et al., 2010). Focusing on patient handling to determine the load on the musculoskeletal system would therefore lead to an underestimate of nurses' total working posture load. Vieira and Kumar (2006) argue that a reduction in peak load may not reduce the risk of lower back injury when the cumulative load increases.

Conclusion

This study showed a significant improvement in body postures after implementation of a training concept consisting of instruction on frequent body postures in nursing, physical exercises, instructions in practical ergonomic work at the bedside and in the bathroom, and reorganization of work environment. As nurses spend a large proportion of time on basic care tasks and these tasks may have the greatest effect on cumulative load, future investigations on prevention and reduction of LBP in nurses may profit by including elements on postural alignment in addition to patient-handling techniques.

Supplementary Data

Supplementary data are available at *Annals of Work Exposures and Health* online.

Funding

No specific funding was received.

Acknowledgements

The authors thank the participating facilities and workers who contributed to the study. The authors declare no conflict of interest relating to the material presented in this article. Its contents, including any opinions and/or conclusions expressed, are solely those of the authors.

References

Alexandre NMC, de Moraes MAA, Corrêa Filho HR *et al.* (2001) Evaluation of a program to reduce back pain in nursing personnel. *Rev Saude Publica*; **35**: 356–61.

Bakker EW, Verhagen AP, van Trijffel E *et al.* (2009) Spinal mechanical load as a risk factor for low back pain: a systematic review of prospective cohort studies. *Spine (Phila Pa 1976)*; **34**: 281–93.

Balague F, Mannion AF, Pellise F *et al.* (2012) Non-specific low back pain. *Lancet*; **379**: 482–91.

Berufsgenossenschaftliches Institut für Arbeitsschutz [Institute for Occupational Safety and Health], BGIA. (1998) *BIA-Report 5/98. Personengebundenes Messsystem zur automatisierten Erfassung von Wirbelsäulenbelastungen bei beruflichen Tätigkeiten* [Personalized measurement system for the automatic measurement of spinal column stress at work]. Sankt Augustin, Germany: Hauptverband der gewerblichen Berufsgenossenschaften [German Federation of Institutions for Statutory Accident Insurance and Prevention].

Best M. (1997) An evaluation of Manutention training in preventing back strain and resultant injuries in nurses. *Safety Sci*; **25**: 207–22.

Bos EH, Krol B, Van Der Star A *et al.* (2006) The effects of occupational interventions on reduction of musculoskeletal symptoms in the nursing profession. *Ergonomics*; **49**: 706–23.

Davis KG, Kotowski SE. (2015) Prevalence of musculoskeletal disorders for nurses in hospitals, long-term care facilities, and home health care: a comprehensive review. *Hum Factors*; **57**: 754–92.

Dawson AP, McLennan SN, Schiller SD *et al.* (2007) Interventions to prevent back pain and back injury in nurses: a systematic review. *Occup Environ Med*; **64**: 642–50.

Dehlin O, Berg S, Andersson GB *et al.* (1981) Effect of physical training and ergonomic counselling on the psychological perception of work and on the subjective assessment of low-back insufficiency. *Scand J Rehabil Med*; **13**: 1–9.

DIN. (2002) *EN 1005-1: Sicherheit von Maschinen—Menschliche Körperliche Leistung—Teil 1: Begriffe* [Safety of machines—human physical performance—part 1: definition of terms]. Berlin, Germany: Beuth Verlag GmbH.

DIN. (2005) *EN 1005-4: Sicherheit von Maschinen—Menschliche Körperliche Leistung—Teil 4: Bewertung von Körperhaltungen und Bewegungen bei der Arbeit an Maschinen* [Safety of machines—human physical performance—part 4: evaluation of postures and movements when working on machines]. Berlin, Germany: Beuth Verlag GmbH.

Ellegast R, Hermanns I, Schiefer C. (2009) Workload assessment in field using the ambulatory CUELA system. In Duffy VG, editor. *Digital human modeling, proceedings*. Berlin, Germany: Springer-Verlag. pp. 221–26.

Engels JA, Landeweerd JA, Kant Y. (1994) An OWAS-based analysis of nurses' working postures. *Ergonomics*; **37**: 909–19.

Engels JA, van der Gulden JWJ, Senden TF *et al.* (1996) Work related risk factors for musculoskeletal complaints in the nursing profession: results of a questionnaire survey. *Occup Environ Med*; **53**: 636–41.

Engels JA, van der Gulden JW, Senden TF *et al.* (1998) The effects of an ergonomic-educational course. Postural load, perceived physical exertion, and biomechanical errors in nursing. *Int Arch Occup Environ Health*; **71**: 336–42.

Engkvist IL, Hjelm EW, Hagberg M *et al.* (2000) Risk indicators for reported over-exertion back injuries among female nursing personnel. *Epidemiology*; **11**: 519–22.

Eriksen W, Bruusgaard D, Knardahl S. (2004) Work factors as predictors of intense or disabling low back pain; a prospective study of nurses' aides. *Occup Environ Med*; **61**: 398–404.

Fanello S, Frampas-Chotard V, Roquelaure Y *et al.* (1999) Evaluation of an educational low back pain prevention program for hospital employees. *Rev Rhum Engl Ed*; **66**: 711–6.

Freitag S, Ellegast R, Dulon M *et al.* (2007) Quantitative measurement of stressful trunk postures in nursing professions. *Ann Occup Hyg*; **51**: 385–95.

Freitag S, Fincke-Junod I, Seddouki R *et al.* (2012) Frequent bending-an underestimated burden in nursing professions. *Ann Occup Hyg*; **56**: 697–707.

Freitag S, Seddouki R, Dulon M *et al.* (2014) The effect of working position on trunk posture and exertion for routine nursing tasks: an experimental study. *Ann Occup Hyg*; **58**: 317–25.

Garg A, Owen B. (1992) Reducing back stress to nursing personnel: an ergonomic intervention in a nursing home. *Ergonomics*; **35**: 1353–75.

Gundewall B, Liljeqvist M, Hansson T. (1993) Primary prevention of back symptoms and absence from work. A prospective randomized study among hospital employees. *Spine (Phila Pa 1976)*; **18**: 587–94.

Hignett S. (2003) Intervention strategies to reduce musculoskeletal injuries associated with handling patients: a systematic review. *Occup Environ Med*; **60**: E6.

Hodder JN, Holmes MW, Keir PJ. (2010) Continuous assessment of work activities and posture in long-term care nurses. *Ergonomics*; **53**: 1097–107.

Holmes MW, Hodder JN, Keir PJ. (2010) Continuous assessment of low back loads in long-term care nurses. *Ergonomics*; **53**: 1108–16.

Holtermann A, Clausen T, Aust B *et al.* (2013) Risk for low back pain from different frequencies, load mass and trunk postures of lifting and carrying among female healthcare workers. *Int Arch Occup Environ Health*; **86**: 463–70.

Horneij E, Hemborg B, Jensen I *et al.* (2001) No significant differences between intervention programmes on neck, shoulder and low back pain: a prospective randomized study among home-care personnel. *J Rehabil Med*; 33: 170–6.

Hoy D, Bain C, Williams G *et al.* (2012) A systematic review of the global prevalence of low back pain. *Arthritis Rheum*; 64: 2028–37.

ISO. (2000) *ISO 11226 ergonomics—evaluation of static working postures.* Geneva, Switzerland: International Organization for Standardisation (IOS).

Jansen JP, Burdorf A, Steyerberg E. (2001) A novel approach for evaluating level, frequency and duration of lumbar posture simultaneously during work. *Scand J Work Environ Health*; 27: 373–80.

Jansen JP, Morgenstern H, Burdorf A. (2004) Dose-response relations between occupational exposures to physical and psychosocial factors and the risk of low back pain. *Occup Environ Med*; 61: 972–9.

Josephson M, Vingård E; Group M-NS. (1998) Workplace factors and care seeking for low-back pain among female nursing personnel. *Scand J Work Environ Health*; 24: 465–72.

Nachemson A. (1975) Towards a better understanding of low-back pain: a review of the mechanics of the lumbar disc. *Rheumatol Rehabil*; 14: 129–43.

Nussbaum MA, Torres N. (2001) Effects of training in modifying working methods during common patient-handling activities. *Int J Ind Ergon*; 27: 33–41.

Occupational Safety and Health Administration. (2009) OSHA 3182-3R 2009. Guidelines for nursing homes – ergonomics for the prevention of musculoskeletal disorders. Available at https://www.osha.gov/ergonomics/guidelines/nursinghome/final_nh_guidelines.html. Accessed 20 September 2015.

Olson MW, Li L, Solomonow M. (2004) Flexion-relaxation response to cyclic lumbar flexion. *Clin Biomech*; 19: 769–76.

Petzäll K, Berglund B, Lundberg C. (2001) The staff's satisfaction with the hospital bed. *J Nurs Manag*; 9: 51–7.

Pohjonen T, Punakallio A, Louhevaara V. (1998) Participatory ergonomics for reducing load and strain in home care work. *Int J Ind Ergon*; 21: 345–52.

Ribeiro DC, Aldabe D, Abbott JH *et al.* (2012) Dose-response relationship between work-related cumulative postural exposure and low back pain: a systematic review. *Ann Occup Hyg*; 56: 684–96.

Ribeiro DC, Sole G, Abbott JH *et al.* (2011) Cumulative postural exposure measured by a novel device: a preliminary study. *Ergonomics*; 54: 858–65.

Roffey DM, Wai EK, Bishop P *et al.* (2010) Causal assessment of awkward occupational postures and low back pain: results of a systematic review. *Spine J*; 10: 89–99.

Smedley J, Egger P, Cooper C *et al.* (1995) Manual handling activities and risk of low back pain in nurses. *Occup Environ Med*; 52: 160–3.

Solomonow M. (2004) Ligaments: a source of work-related musculoskeletal disorders. *J Electromyogr Kinesiol*; 14: 49–60.

Solomonow M, Baratta RV, Banks A *et al.* (2003) Flexion–relaxation response to static lumbar flexion in males and females. *Clin Biomech*; 18: 273–79.

Tullar JM, Brewer S, Amick BC 3rd *et al.* (2010) Occupational safety and health interventions to reduce musculoskeletal symptoms in the health care sector. *J Occup rehabil*; 20: 199–219.

Videman T, Rauhala H, Asp S *et al.* (1989) Patient-handling skill, back injuries, and back pain. An intervention study in nursing. *Spine (Phila Pa 1976)*; 14: 148–56.

Vieira ER, Kumar S. (2006) Cut-points to prevent low back injury due to force exertion at work. *Work*; 27: 75–87.

Wai EK, Roffey DM, Bishop P *et al.* (2010) Causal assessment of occupational bending or twisting and low back pain: results of a systematic review. *Spine J*; 10: 76–88.

Wilke HJ, Neef P, Caimi M *et al.* (1999) New in vivo measurements of pressures in the intervertebral disc in daily life. *Spine (Phila Pa 1976)*; 24: 755–62.

Yassi A, Lockhart K. (2013) Work-relatedness of low back pain in nursing personnel: a systematic review. *Int J Occup Environ Health*; 19: 223–44.

Yip VY. (2004) New low back pain in nurses: work activities, work stress and sedentary lifestyle. *J Adv Nurs*; 46: 430–40.

Abkürzungsverzeichnis

ACGIH	American Conference of Governmental Industrial Hygienists		**HAL**	Hand Activity Level (Aktivitätsgrade der Hand)
AL	Action Level		**HR**	Hazard Ratio
AMSTAR-R	Assessment of Multiple Systematic Reviews – Revised		**HWS**	Halswirbelsäule
			ICC	Intraclass correlation
AU	Arbeitsunfähigkeit		**KTS**	Karpaltunnelsyndrom
BGW	Berufsgenossenschaft für Gesundheitsdienst und Wohlfahrtspflege		**LWS**	Lendenwirbelsäule
			MOOSE	Meta-analysis of Observational Studies in Epidemiology
BK	Berufskrankheit		**MSB**	Muskel-Skelett-Beschwerden
BMI	Body-Mass-Index		**MSE**	Muskel-Skelett-Erkrankungen
CCA	Corrected Covered Area		**NLG**	Nervenleitgeschwindigkeitstest
COPSOQ	Copenhagen Psychosocial Questionnaire		**NIOSH**	National Institute of Occupational Safety and Health
CTD	Cumulative Trauma Disorders		**PEROSH**	Partnership for European Research in Occupational Safety andHealth, Arbeitsgruppe Clearinghouse of Systematic Reviews
CUELA	Computerunterstützte Erfassung und Langzeitanalyse von Muskel-Skelett-Belastungen			
CVcare	Competenzzentrum Epidemiologie und Versorgungsforschung bei Pflegeberufen		**RSI**	Repetitive Strain Injury
			RR	Relatives Risiko
			SES	Sozioökonomischer Status
DALY	Disability Adjusted Life Years		**SPA**	Sozialpädagogische Assistenz
GuK	Gesundheits- und Krankenpflege		**SR**	Systematisches Review
			TLV	Threshold Limit Value

Abbildungsverzeichnis